Turmeric
& Healing Spices

Remedies for health and well-being

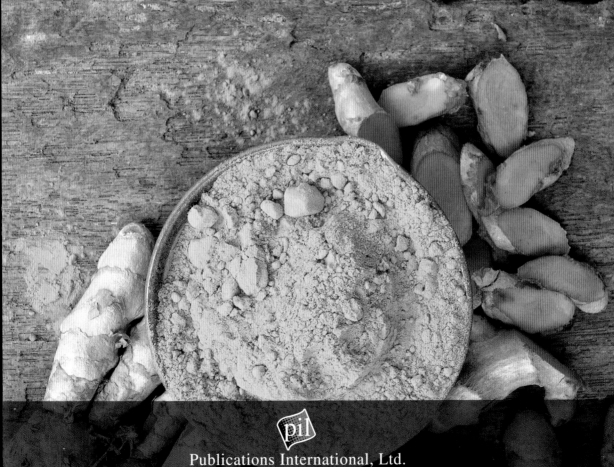

pil

Publications International, Ltd.

MW01078387

Written by: Lisa Brooks

Photography: Shutterstock.com and WikiMedia Commons

Copyright © 2019 Publications International, Ltd. All rights reserved. This book may not be reproduced or quoted in whole or in part by any means whatsoever without written permission from:

Louis Weber, CEO
Publications International, Ltd.
8140 Lehigh Avenue
Morton Grove, IL 60053

Permission is never granted for commercial purposes.

ISBN: 978-1-64030-866-4

Manufactured in China.

8 7 6 5 4 3 2 1

This publication is only intended to provide general information. The information is specifically not intended to be substitute for medical diagnosis or treatment by your physician or other healthcare professional. You should always consult your own physician or other healthcare professionals about any medical questions, diagnosis, or treatment. (Products vary among manufacturers. Please check labels carefully to confirm that the products you use are appropriate for your condition.)

The information obtained by you from this publication should not be relied upon for any personal, nutritional, or medical decision. You should consult an appropriate professional for specific advice tailored to your specific situation. PIL makes no representation or warranties, express or implied, with respect to your use of this information.

In no event shall PIL or its affiliates or advertisers be liable for any direct, indirect, punitive, incidental, special, or consequential damages, or any damages whatsoever including, without limitation, damages for personal injury, death, damage to property or loss of profits, arising out of or in any way connected with the use of any of the above-referenced information or otherwise arising out of use of this publication.

Table of Contents

Introduction — 4

Turmeric — 6
Ancient Roots — 8
What Is Ayurvedic Medicine? — 10
Turmeric Today — 12
Curcumin — 14
Turmeric as Medicine: an Overview — 16
Inflammation — 18
An Antioxidant Effect — 20
Arthritis — 22
Aging — 26
Alzheimer's Disease — 28
Depression — 30
High Cholesterol — 32
Heart Health — 34
Diabetes — 36
Cancer and Cancer Treatment — 38
Digestive Issues — 42
Inflammatory Bowel Diseases — 44
Skin Problems — 46
Hay Fever — 48
Taking Turmeric — 50
Cautions — 52
Recipes — 54

Other Healing Spices — 64
Ajwain — 66
Allspice — 68
Asafetida — 72
Black Pepper — 74
Caraway — 78
Cardamom — 82
Cayenne Pepper — 86
Chia Seed — 90
Celery Seed — 92
Cinnamon — 94
Cloves — 98
Coriander — 102
Cumin — 106
Dill Seed — 110
Fennel — 114
Garlic — 118
Ginger — 140
Ginseng — 146
Horseradish — 148
Mustard — 154
Nutmeg and Mace — 160
Paprika — 164
Poppy Seed — 168
Saffron — 172
Sesame Seed — 176
Star Anise — 182
Sumac — 186
Vanilla — 188

Introduction

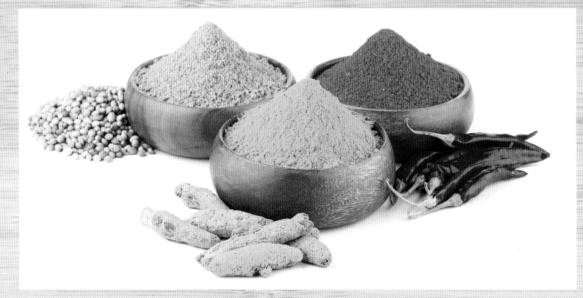

We grew up hearing "you are what you eat" and thinking of certain foods as healthy or unhealthy, nutritious or not. But we don't usually spend much time thinking about the spices that season our foods and the health benefits they might bring us. However, the roots, seeds, stems, and bark of plants, in the forms of spices, can also affect our health, as can the leaves of plants in the form of herbs.

One of those spices, turmeric, an essential flavoring in South Asian cuisine, has been receiving a lot of fresh buzz lately for its healing properties—although as you'll find out, it has been used medically for thousands of years! Turmeric and its key component, curcumin, are available as supplements in oil, pill, powder form, and more. You've no doubt heard of the concept of a "superfood." Turmeric could be labeled a "superspice" in terms of the ways it is credited with supporting health. But does it live up to the hype?

In this book, we'll look at the wide array of conditions that turmeric is purported to help treat, including arthritis, diabetes, high cholesterol, and cancer. You'll find out about how you might use it to boost your health or aid recovery. But don't stop with turmeric—find out about other seasonings such as ginger, garlic, horseradish, coriander and more, and how they have been used to treat health conditions.

We tend to think of healthy foods as bland or boring ones. But you can combine tasty food with health benefits through the use of herbs and spices! Spices can also be used in healing teas, in supplement form, and in essential oil forms.

Essential Oils

In this book, you'll find some suggestions for using certain spices in their essential oil form, topically or with diffusers. Essential oils can be purchased in health stores, some grocery stores, and of course online. Their easy availability and the fact that they are distilled directly from plants may make cautionary guidelines seem unnecessary—after all, there are no FDA warnings or lists of side effects on their labels—but you should never underestimate the capacity this natural pharmacy has for both beneficial and harmful results. Essential oils contain powerful chemical compounds. Misuse via direct topical application or ingestion can result in serious harm. Even when using essential oils via diffusion, consider the dilution rate and size of the room. Can the oils disperse readily? How long will the exposure be? Prolonged exposure (over one hour) to relatively high levels of essential oil vapor may lead to nausea, headache, or feeling "spaced out." If you find yourself feeling like this, get some fresh air right away. Brief exposure is better.

Infants and toddlers are more sensitive to the potency of essential oils. What's safe and pleasant for adults may be overwhelming for young children. The recipes in this book are not intended for children. You should never ingest essential oils. There are some instances where practitioners will recommend the ingestion of small, diluted amounts to address specific conditions, but you should never do this without the guidance of a qualified professional.

When applying essential oils to the skin, always dilute them with a carrier oil. As you increase the ratio of essential oil to carrier oil, you run a greater risk of an adverse dermal reaction. Rubbing just a few drops of most essential oils directly onto the skin could easily amount to ingesting the equivalent of 10 cups of herb tea all at once! In addition to irritating or even burning your skin, you could damage your liver and kidneys, which must detoxify large amounts of essential oils once they enter the blood stream.

While many oils are generally well-tolerated by most individuals when applied via massage in a carrier oil, others are best avoided. Be especially careful with these following essential oils, as they are known to be dermal irritants: Cinnamon bark or leaf, cloves, cumin, and ginger. Cumin is also a photosensitizer; when using the essential oil, avoid prolonged exposure to sunlight for 24 hours.

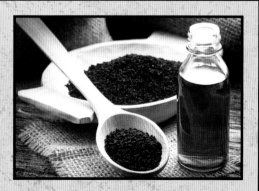

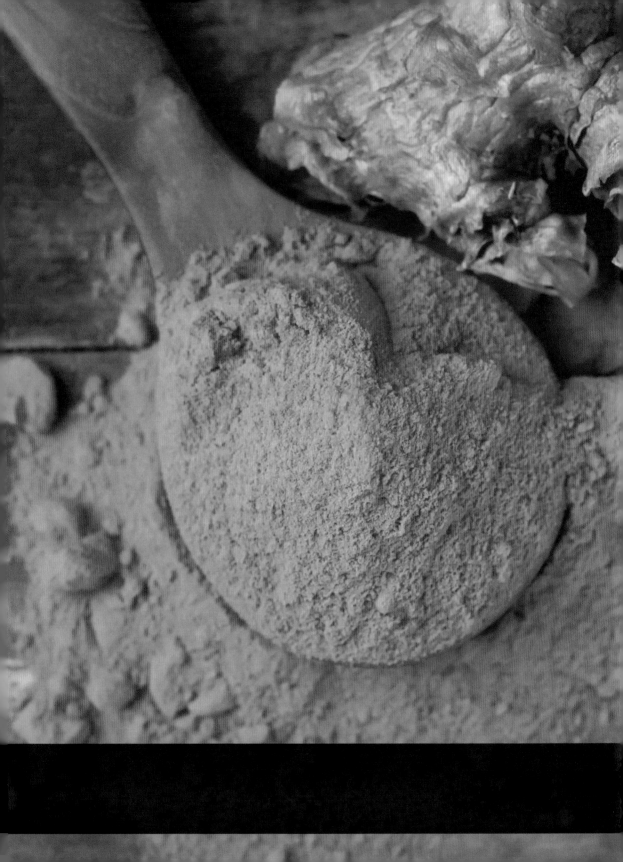

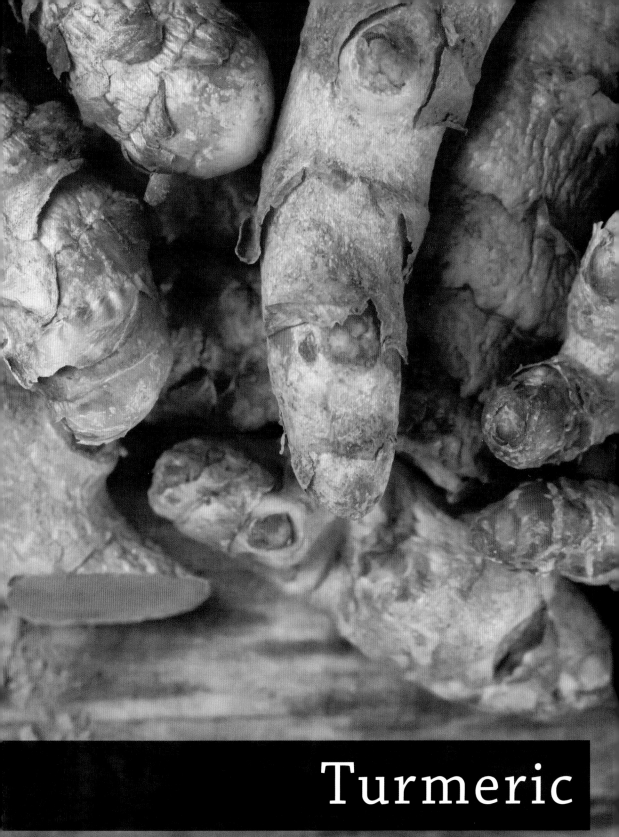

Turmeric

Ancient Roots

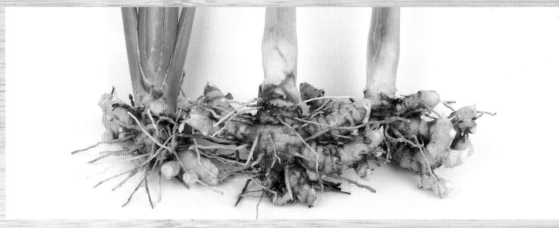

C. aromatica may be the wild ancestor of turmeric.

Some food crops have been cultivated by humans so long that it is no longer clear when they were first domesticated or where they originated. Turmeric (aptly named *Curcuma domestica*) is one such plant. It is a sterile triploid—it produces no seeds and can't be found in the wild. Its closest relative may be C. *aromatica*, which is native to India. It seems probable that turmeric comes from southern or western India, but this has yet to be proven. A number of other wild species of *Curcuma* can be found throughout the southeastern region of Asia.

Humans have been growing and harvesting turmeric for at least 4,000 years—probably longer. One of its first uses may have been as a vegetable dye for cloth. We know that the Vedic culture of India used turmeric as both a culinary and medicinal spice and for religious purposes at least this long ago thanks to oral histories that made their way into the written record. Its vibrant yellow color suggested an affinity with the sun, and it was probably due to this that it became associated with sun-worshipping rituals.

In the Atharva Veda (a collection of Vedic scriptures compiled in Sanskrit roughly 3,000 years ago) turmeric makes a prominent appearance as *haridra*. Even in those ancient times, it was noted as a multipurpose panacea. A mixture of haridra powder and honey was taken to improve memory. Mixed with ghee, it was applied to snake bites. It was thought to help counteract graying hair. A significant number of remedies for skin diseases included haridra in their list of ingredients. From these origins, the root became a common ingredient in Ayurvedic medicine. By 250 BC, the famous Ayurvedic physician Sushruta noted in his *Compendium* that an ointment of turmeric would relieve food poisoning and heal wounds.

An Ayurvedic Powerhouse

Ayurvedic healing practices used turmeric to purify the blood, treat epilepsy, ease diarrhea, treat respiratory ailments, fight infection, and treat urinary tract issues. It was used as a paste, dried powder, and in juice form. The Ayurvedic system considers turmeric to be a balancing agent that helps the human system achieve harmony among the three doshas. It continues to play a role in ayurvedic healing.

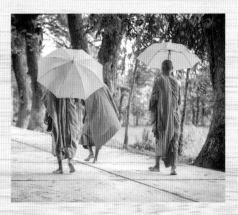

Turmeric dyes cloth a warm shade of yellow-orange, although it fades quickly. It is one of the sources some Buddhist monks use to color their robes.

From India to the World

As turmeric grew in importance within India, it also grew in geographic scope. It traveled via caravan west to the Middle East and Asia Minor. By 710 BC, a Babylonian king was growing turmeric in his royal garden. The Roman writer Pliny gave it a passing mention in the first century AD. Arab traders introduced it to the eastern coast of Africa by the eighth century. Turmeric's arrival in China is hard to pinpoint, but it is known that it was being traded there by AD 600. The plant seems to have had high value in Polynesian cultures: as European explorers began arriving on the shores of south Pacific islands in the eighteenth century, they often noted residents that grew turmeric and used it on their skin.

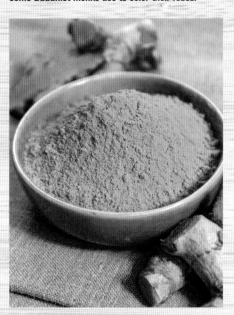

Oldest Dish on the Planet?

In 2013, archaeologists examined the residue found on human dental remains and within pots from Farmana, a site roughly 100 miles northwest of New Delhi. The artifacts and teeth were over 4,000 years old. The residue included a number of spices, including turmeric, garlic, and ginger. Sound familiar? That's right—the Indian dish we know as curry is older than some of the Egyptian pyramids.

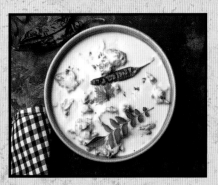

What Is Ayurvedic Medicine?

An ancient healing tradition, Ayurvedic medicine is still practiced throughout the Indian subcontinent and is enjoying a burgeoning popularity in the West. In the ancient Indian language Sanskrit, Ayurveda means "the science of longevity" and is sometimes translated more broadly as "the science of life." The system seeks to restore harmony and balance to the body, mind, and spirit through a system of diet, herbal medicine, massage, purification, and lifestyle discipline.

A Healthy Lifestyle

In Ayurvedic medicine, the patient is active in his or her own preventative therapy. In this sense, Ayurveda is much more concerned with health than with disease—with the healthy person rather than with the unhealthy patient. Although one of the features that makes Ayurveda so popular today is its "holistic" approach, the truth is Ayurvedic medicine is firmly grounded in empirical observation and scientific theory. And while its ancient development and practice are not entirely devoid of magical charms and incantations, some of the earliest treatises on Ayurveda are remarkably rational and scientific.

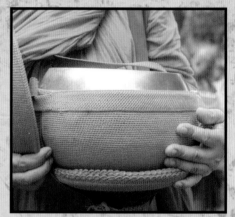

Diverse Beginnings

Scholars of Indology cannot determine the exact origins of Ayurveda, but we can see how many different traditions combined to create it over the millennia. The magical, religious lore of early Indian civilizations, the more empirical and practical approach of the so-called wandering ascetics, the medical traditions of the early Buddhist monks, and possible additions from neighboring traditions all work together to provide the basis of what we know as Ayurveda.

Out of these traditions emerges a system eventually codified in the two great Ayurvedic medical treatises—*Caraka Samhita* and *Susruta Samhita*. Although these two works, which provide the basis for the entire system, are considered Hindu, the information in them clearly developed over the centuries with significant help from the Buddhists and other religious and secular traditions.

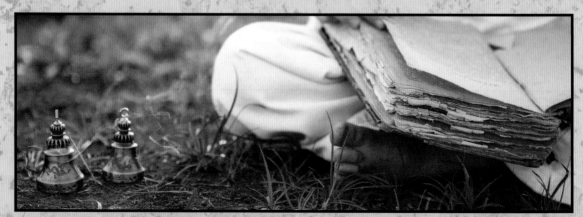

Doshas and the Understanding of Disease

Perhaps no other culture influenced the early medical lore that was to become Ayurveda more than the Buddhist monks. About the middle of the fifth century BC, many Buddhist ascetics began to organize into spiritual communities called sanghas. As the sangha population stabilized, the monks and nuns began to standardize and codify all the medical information they had gathered. Much of this material can be found in the *Vinaya Pitaka* of the Buddhist Pali Canon, devoted to the code of conduct for the Buddhist monk.

The chapter on medicine represents the earliest form of Buddhist healing and closely parallels some of the information that would later be set down in the *Caraka Samhita* and the *Susruta Samhita*. Once written, this Buddhist "order of things" became the first step toward an Indian medical system. The Buddha identified the causes of disease as falling into one of the following categories:

- a change of season
- past actions (karma)
- unusual or excessive activities
- violent, external actions (being robbed or attacked)

Sramanic and Buddhist healers believed that humans represent or reflect the whole of nature—a belief also found in the Vedas. In other words, humans are microcosms of the universe, containing the same elements that make up all of creation. These elements—space (or ether), air, fire, water, and earth—are combined into three biological forces, or *doshas*, in humans—*vata*, *pitta*, and *kapha*.

- Vata is space and air.
- Pitta is fire and water.
- Kapha is water and earth.

The doshas came to be seen as responsible for all the functions of our bodies and minds. English has no adequate translation for the word dosha. Although you'll often see them referred to as air, fire, and water, respectively, or (less delicately) wind, bile, and phlegm, the concept of the dosha is more than that; for example, vata has wind-like qualities, but it is not simply wind.

The Buddhist canon, and later Ayurvedic medicine, views disease as a disruption of the doshas. Since all disease stems from a disruption in the doshas, treatment must begin to return the body to a state of doshic harmony. Ayurvedic physicians use diet, herbs, and cleansing techniques to counteract the manifestation of disease in the body.

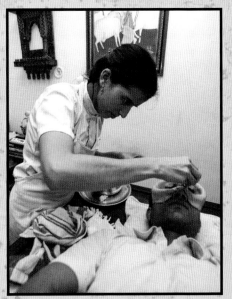

An Ayurvedic clinic in India

Turmeric Today

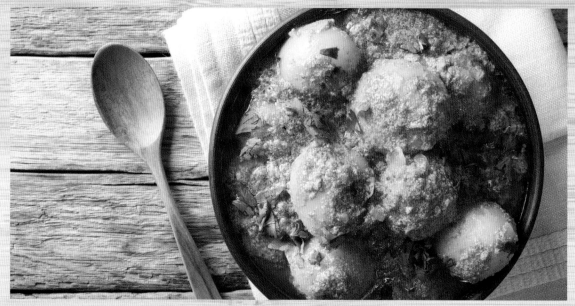

Potatoes in curry sauce highlight the tasty use of turmeric.

In the 1747 book *The Art of Cookery Made Plain and Easy*, author Hannah Glasse included a page describing "India pickle." The recipe for this exotic Eastern condiment was the first time a Western English recipe called for turmeric. The spice made its way to Europe in the mid-17th century, due to the British colonization of India and trading through the British East India Trading Company. Later editions of Glasse's cookbook included a recipe for a curry dish, and in 1831, the cookbook *Virginia Housewife*, by Mary Randolph, became the first American cookbook to feature curry.

As the spicy dishes gained popularity in the West, Indian merchants began selling powdered mixtures of curry spices—including turmeric—to British traders who carried them home. The clever merchants not only marketed these spices as flavorful additions to recipes, but also as cure-alls for whatever ailed their customers.

While the British travelers may have found the claims of turmeric's healing properties quite interesting—and there's no denying that turmeric has been used for medicinal purposes in many parts of the world for centuries—over time, the golden spice was much less likely to be found in a medicine cabinet than on a dinner plate. Not that anyone can complain: Its bold flavor and distinctive hue add punch not only to curries, but also to many other dishes, and its tendency to stain any substance it encounters makes it a great alternative to artificial coloring in foods like cake, ice cream, and beverages.

Certainly, the culinary versatility of turmeric has given it a well-deserved place in many kitchens. But recently, the ancient medicinal benefits of this colorful spice have been reexamined, and a whole new generation of people are embracing turmeric as more than simply a pantry staple.

And it's no wonder: Americans spend billions of dollars every year on natural and alternative medicinal remedies, which include everything from acupuncture to meditation to probiotics. While it can be easy to dismiss such therapies as nothing more than placebos, research and anecdotal evidence often back up their beneficial effects. Such is the case with turmeric. While our ancient forebears already knew that this spice could be used for treating cuts and burns or for improving digestion, modern studies are showing that turmeric may be useful for so much more.

One area in which the spice has shown great promise is in the treatment of depression. Several studies have shown that a combination of antidepressant medication and turmeric supplements lead to a significantly greater reduction in symptoms compared to antidepressants alone. In fact, turmeric's ability to lessen depression is so powerful that even on its own, it has been shown to reduce symptoms almost as well as Prozac! With around 13 percent of Americans taking antidepressants—which can result in side effects like weight gain, insomnia, dizziness, or even a worsening of depression—turmeric's uplifting influence is worth noting.

But treating depression is just the tip of the iceberg for this spice, which has been shown to be effective at easing the pain of arthritis, relieving symptoms of indigestion, heartburn, and irritable bowel syndrome, and preventing heart attacks in bypass patients. Encouraged by turmeric's obvious medicinal benefits, curious researchers have continued to study the spice, which shows promise for a myriad of ailments, including liver disorders, Crohn's disease, cancer, and Alzheimer's disease. Its anti-inflammatory properties also make it a good spice to have on hand for anyone who wants to avoid over-the-counter painkillers, or for those who struggle with acne.

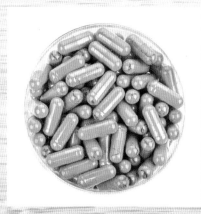

Supplement pills

So what makes turmeric such a potent and beneficial spice? It all comes down to turmeric's golden-hued active ingredient: curcumin.

Curcumin

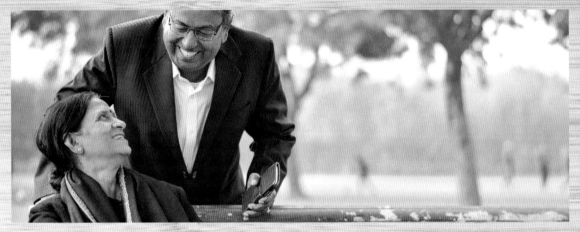

Rates of Alzheimer's disease are lower in India than in many other countries.

The terms "turmeric" and "curcumin" are sometimes used interchangeably. But while turmeric is the plant that is used to create the spice enjoyed by Indian-food aficionados, curcumin is a compound found within turmeric that gives the spice its yellow color and many health benefits. Recent research has suggested that this substance is an effective anti-inflammatory and antioxidant agent, and it is also showing promise in the treatment of diabetes and certain cancers. The compound may actually have the ability to block an enzyme that is responsible for turning environmental toxins into carcinogens within the body. This may make curcumin a vitally important substance for cancer researchers in years to come.

Known as a "curcuminoid," curcumin is the principal active ingredient in turmeric, which also contains carbohydrates, protein, minerals, fiber, fat, essential oils, and water. This means that curcumin, while the most powerful substance in the golden spice, makes up only about 3 percent of the spice on average. The other curcuminoids in turmeric—including the tongue-twisting substances "demethoxycurcumin" and "bisdemethoxycurcumin"—make up even less of the total compounds.

In a diet where turmeric is regularly consumed, this low percentage of curcumin may not be a problem. For instance, in India, where it's customary to consume turmeric many times a week, incidents of Alzheimer's disease are much lower than in other parts of the world. Researchers speculate that curcumin's anti-inflammatory properties protect the brains of those who regularly consume it. But in America, and many other parts of the world, turmeric is not always a regular part of our diets. It can be harder to benefit from curcumin's effects when it makes up such a small part of the turmeric spice and we eat it so infrequently.

And there's another caveat to consider when it comes to curcumin consumption: The substance has poor bioavailability, meaning it is difficult for humans to absorb it. If it is ingested on its own, curcumin is quickly metabolized and eliminated, with very little of its beneficial goodness left behind. So what can be done to counter these issues and make sure we reap the benefits of this spicy substance?

Fortunately, the issues of curcumin ingestion and absorption have some simple solutions. Perhaps the most obvious remedy to ensure a beneficial amount of curcumin in your diet is to eat curries many times a week. (And why not? Curry is delicious!) But not all of us want to overhaul our diets that drastically. While books, cooking shows, and the internet are teeming with a huge variety of turmeric recipes—everything from soups, stews, and roasts to pickles, tea, and ice cream—there's an even easier way to add the spice into your diet: supplements.

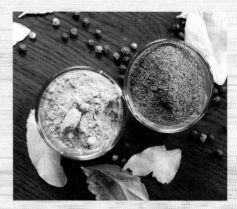

Black pepper helps with turmeric absorption.

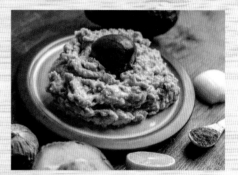

Foods such as avocado with a high percentage of healthy fats may help you absorb curcumin.

Curcumin is often extracted from turmeric and used to make tablets, capsules, or liquid that can easily be consumed daily—no cooking required! But what about curcumin's poor bioavailability? Researchers have discovered a solution for that as well, and the answer comes from another staple you no doubt have in your pantry: black pepper. Peperine, the substance responsible for the pungency of black pepper, increases the absorption of curcumin by an astounding 2,000 percent. So if you're eating your curcumin in curries or other foods, be sure to include black pepper with your meal. And if you're using supplements, look for one that includes both curcumin and peperine, to be sure that the benefits aren't wasted.

Another curcumin characteristic to note is its fat solubility. To make it even easier for your body to absorb the substance, it can help to take supplements with foods with a high fat content, such as olive oil, avocado, or cheese. If you're eating your curcumin in food, you'll want a bit of fat along with the black pepper, to ensure the best possible absorption of this potent compound.

Turmeric as Medicine: an Overview

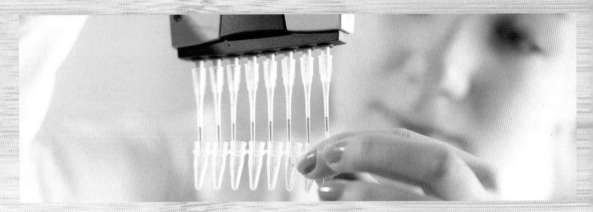

Considering all of the potential turmeric has shown—not to mention its already-proven benefits —there are some who call the golden spice the most effective nutritional supplement on Earth. Of course it's delicious when used in curries, soups, and teas, but turmeric is so much more than simply a way to flavor our food—it's also a potent medicine.

Turmeric has been found to be especially beneficial in two ways: as an anti-inflammatory, and as an antioxidant. These two properties give the spice an ability to help fight, treat, or prevent a variety of ailments. In fact, some studies have found the spice to be just as powerful as pharmaceuticals, making it even more attractive to those who wish to avoid drugs, but still need relief from pain, illness, or depression.

We'll delve into turmeric's anti-inflammatory and antioxidant properties in a moment, but first, let's talk about a few of the other amazing ways the spice has been making waves in the medical world. For instance, research has shown that curcumin can boost something called "brain-derived neurotropic factor," or BDNF, which is a growth hormone in the brain. BDFN helps to create and multiply neurons in the brain, and form connections between neural pathways. Decreased levels of this important hormone have been linked to disorders including Alzheimer's disease, depression, and other brain diseases. But curcumin increases levels of BDFN, which can help to delay or even reverse some diseases or age-related decreases in brain function.

Heart disease is another issue that turmeric is being used to address, as curcumin has been shown to improve the function of the lining of blood vessels, lowing blood pressure and preventing blood clots. What's more, if taken before and after heart surgery, curcumin has been proven to reduce the risk of surgery-related heart attack by 65 percent. Studies have shown that the supplement improves blood vessel function as well as exercise, and one study even showed that curcumin worked as well as the popular drug Atorvastatin.

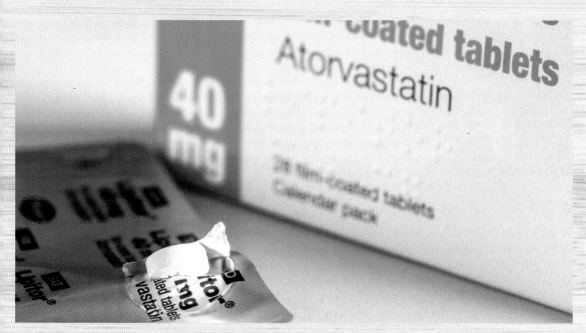

Atorvastatin is often used to treat high cholesterol.

Some of the most exciting turmeric research has studied its effects on cancer cells and tumors. Curcumin has been shown to influence the growth, development, and spread of cancer cells at a molecular level, with an ability to kill the cells and reduce both the spread of the disease—known as metastasis—and the growth of new blood vessels in tumors, stifling their growth. Research suggests that taking daily turmeric supplements can stabilize certain kinds of cancer, including colon and prostate. But perhaps even more promising is turmeric's potential to prevent cancer from occurring in the first place. Studies in people with a high risk for colon cancer have shown that a daily turmeric supplement reduces the chance of cancerous lesions by 40 percent. Although more research is needed to confirm that turmeric can treat cancer rather than just prevent it, medical professionals hope that one day the spice can be used alongside conventional treatments as a cancer killer.

Turmeric's benefits for those suffering from depression have been especially well researched, with curcumin demonstrating an effectiveness similar to Prozac. Since depression has been linked to a reduced level of BDFN in the brain, curcumin's ability to boost this hormone can reduce the changes that occur in those with low levels of BDFN. There is also evidence that curcumin can raise levels of the brain neurotransmitters serotonin and dopamine, which are linked to mood and happiness.

Other conditions that may benefit from the medicinal effects of turmeric include high cholesterol, Crohn's disease, diabetes, skin rashes, and kidney and liver problems. Possible treatments are looking very promising, thanks to this versatile spice.

Inflammation

Turmeric's anti-inflammatory properties are one of the characteristics that make it so effective against many different ailments. But what, exactly, is inflammation, and why are anti-inflammatories important?

It may be surprising to learn that inflammation is actually quite a beneficial part of the immune system. When we are injured or have an infection, inflammation is the body's way of signaling the immune system to begin healing and repairing damaged tissue, or to fight off harmful invaders like viruses and bacteria. When an injury or infection occurs, blood vessels dilate, blood flow increases, and white blood cells rush to the area to begin the healing process. This can result in swelling, redness, and pain, but without this important physiological response, infections could easily become deadly and wounds would never heal.

This short-term inflammation helps to keep us healthy and the body's systems running smoothly. But when an inflammatory response lasts too long, or if it occurs in an area where it's not needed, inflammation becomes a problem. In fact, scientists believe that unchecked inflammation may be to blame for a myriad of chronic diseases, including heart disease, cancer, and many degenerative disorders.

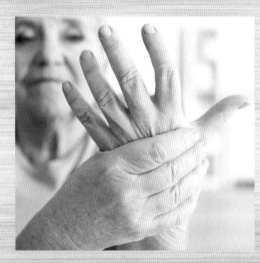

Inflammation is also the cause of autoimmune disorders like rheumatoid arthritis and lupus. Autoimmune disorders occur when the immune system mistakes a benign part of the body—like the skin or joints—for a foreign invader, and sends inflammation to attack. The factors behind autoimmune inflammation are largely unknown, although researchers suspect that genetics, environmental influences, and diet can all play a role. Women are also twice as likely to have an autoimmune disorder as men.

But it's a different type of inflammation—called chronic inflammation—that researchers believe can contribute to illnesses like heart disease and cancer. Chronic inflammation is a consistent, low-grade inflammation that often has no symptoms, but can show up as a slight rise in immune system markers in a blood test. This chronic inflammation causes white blood cells to aimlessly gather, with nowhere to go and nothing to do.

Eventually, these bored white blood cells may decide to attack healthy tissues and cells. For instance, chronic inflammation in the blood vessels can lead to a buildup of plaque, which can eventually form clots that block blood flow and lead to heart attacks or strokes.

Obviously, inflammation is not always a beneficial process. But treating it—and, perhaps more importantly, preventing it—is certainly possible. Anti-inflammatory drugs like aspirin and ibuprofen can target temporary bouts of inflammation, and many doctors and nutritionists recommend an anti-inflammatory diet—which is low in saturated fats, sugars, and refined carbohydrates, and high in fruits, vegetables, lean meats, and healthy fats—to keep chronic inflammation at bay. But there's another dietary addition that may have an even more powerful effect: turmeric.

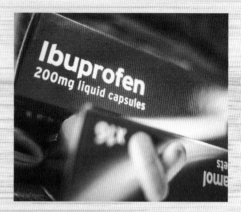
Steady use of ibuprofen can cause unwanted side effects.

The curcumin in turmeric blocks the inflammatory cytokines and enzymes that are responsible for conditions like arthritis and bursitis, and which, if left unchecked, can also cause chronic inflammation. Turmeric has been shown to not only relieve the pain and inflammation caused by arthritis, but in some cases, it has even been proven to work better than nonsteroidal anti-inflammatory drugs (NSAIDs) like ibuprofen or the prescription-strength drug diclofenac.

Even better, when taken regularly, turmeric supplements can control chronic inflammation, preventing aimless white blood cells from organizing into a targeted attack against healthy tissues. And of course, turmeric can do all of this with a much lower risk of side effects than NSAIDs, which can often cause stomach upset, liver and kidney problems, or high blood pressure.

Since scientists believe that inflammation plays a role in many disorders—including some of the biggest killers in the U.S. like heart disease, cancer, and diabetes—turmeric's anti-inflammatory properties make it a potent weapon to add to your healthy-living arsenal.

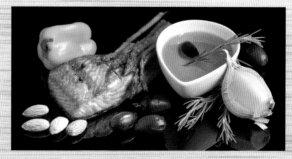
The Mediterranean diet is often recommended to decrease inflammation.

Remedies for health and well-being 19

An Antioxidant Effect

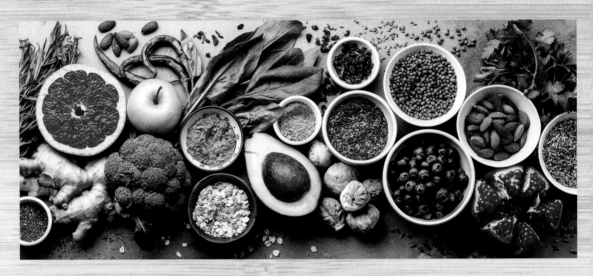

Think of a commercial for a "healthy" product—maybe a juice, or a smoothie, or a vitamin supplement. Chances are, the word "antioxidant" shows up at some point during the sales pitch, immediately conjuring an idea of a nutritional powerhouse that delivers all kinds of vital benefits to the body. But for all the times we've heard this buzzword thrown around, how much do we actually know about antioxidants? What exactly are they, and why are they considered such a good thing?

As the name suggests, antioxidants fight a process within the cells of the body called oxidation. In this process, our cells are constantly undergoing chemical reactions in which electrons in sugar, fatty acid, and amino acid molecules are shifted around and added to oxygen molecules. This creates unstable particles known as "free radicals," which can also form when we are exposed to things like ultraviolet light, pollution, or cigarette smoke. Once free radicals form, they can combine with other molecules, including our DNA, and damage them. Free radicals can even create a chain reaction, turning damaged molecules into more free radicals, which can damage more cells, and so on.

Antioxidants can be helpful during this oxidation process by providing extra electrons to free radicals. When an antioxidant offers an electron to a free radical, it becomes oxidized itself, effectively neutralizing the free radical and preventing cell damage. But surprisingly, just like inflammation, free radicals aren't always harmful. These molecules are used to convert air and food into energy for the body, and the immune system uses free radicals to fight off bacteria and infections. So it's important to have a balance between free radicals and antioxidants.

However, if this balance is upturned, and free radicals begin to outnumber antioxidants, it results in what is called "oxidative stress." And if we're exposed to more oxidative stress than our bodies can handle, free radicals can cause serious damage, and may play a part in the development of many different illnesses and disorders. For instance, oxidation of DNA may eventually lead to cancer, while oxidation of cholesterol makes it even more damaging to blood vessels and results in heart disease. Free radicals are even believed to speed up the aging process—a scary thought for most of us!

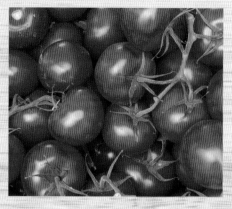

Lycopene gives both watermelons and tomatoes their red color.

Antioxidants include substances like beta-carotene, found in carrots and sweet potatoes; lutein, found in leafy greens; lycopene, found in tomatoes and watermelon; and of course, curcuminoids, found in turmeric. Fruits, vegetables, coffee, and tea are great sources of antioxidants, but turmeric has a unique property that gives it extra antioxidant punch. The spice has been found to boost the antioxidant capacity of the body by not only blocking free radicals directly, but also by increasing the body's own antioxidant enzymes. This two-sided attack makes turmeric an especially potent free radical fighter and a double threat to oxidative stress.

While antioxidants like vitamins C and E are well-known and easily found in many foods, turmeric's abilities far outweigh these common sources. The antioxidants in turmeric are at least five times stronger than those in vitamin E, and ten times stronger than vitamin C. These potent antioxidant properties can help stave off heart disease, cancer, and other chronic illnesses, and can help prevent premature aging and age-related disorders.

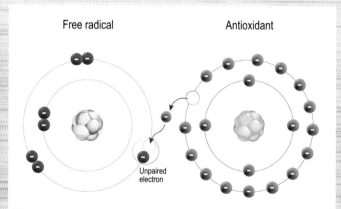

Free radical

Antioxidant

Unpaired electron

The important thing to remember with antioxidants is that too much of any single supplement can tilt the balance between antioxidants and free radicals in the wrong direction. For this reason, it is best to avoid synthetic supplements and instead ingest plenty of natural antioxidant sources, including the amazing golden spice, turmeric.

Arthritis

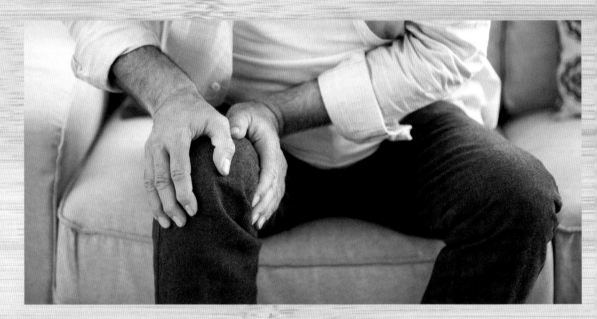

It's a common tabloid headline—"Miracle Cure for Arthritis!" Arthritis is the kind of disease that's a perfect target for such scams. It's not well understood, so anything goes when it comes to theories and treatments. And arthritis often strikes older folks—favorite targets of charlatans.

If you suffer from arthritis, you know how desperate you can get for relief. You may feel you have nothing to lose by trying an alleged cure. After all, your own doctor may not be able to offer much relief, and what medicines there are—primarily nonsteroidal anti-inflammatory drugs and steroids—have limited benefits and may cause some unpleasant side effects, as well.

Most important for scam artists, arthritis is unpredictable, with natural flare-ups and remissions. This, of course, makes it very difficult for patients to know for sure if any improvement is the result of a specific treatment or just a normal remission. Arthritis is a natural for the placebo effect, when the patient's expectation that a treatment will work can actually result in improvement.

Many Diseases, One Name

Arthritis isn't really a single disease at all. It's a term used to describe more than 100 disorders known collectively as rheumatic diseases. Although the Greek word arthritis literally means "joint inflammation," even this classic symptom isn't present in all types.

Stages of knee Osteoarthritis

Stage I	Stage II	Stage III	Stage IV
Doubtful	Mild	Moderate	Severe

Osteoarthritis

Take osteoarthritis (OA), the most common form of arthritis. It often involves no inflammation. OA is a degenerative joint disease; weight-bearing joints simply wear themselves out. This is a stereotypical condition of old age, but it's not uncommon in the younger crowd. It's particularly common among athletes (baseball players, golfers, tennis players), typists, pianists—anyone who pounds joints.

It may start, for whatever reason (maybe heredity), with the thinning out of cartilage between joints. Eventually, wear and tear destroys the cartilage. This creates painful bone-on-bone rubbing. If you're overweight, you're more likely to develop OA, because there's more stress and strain on your joints, particularly your knees. Research shows that, conversely, if you lose excess weight—at least 11 pounds, according to one study of overweight middle-aged women—you can cut in half your risk of developing OA of the knee.

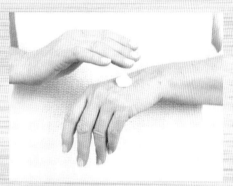

Exercise such as tai chi may help reduce pain and increase mobility.

Over-the-counter pain medication may help, as well as stronger pain medication prescribed by a doctor and cortisone injections. Exercise—particularly the gentle moves of tai chi—may help, as well as physical therapy. Eventually a person may need joint replacement.

A number of supplements are recommended for those suffering from arthritis, and you may want to ask your doctor for recommendations on those that would fit into your treatment plan and that would not interact badly with other medications you are taking. Avocado-soybean unsaponifiables, a nutritional supplement that mixes together avocado and soybean oils, has been recommended for stalling joint damage based on good results in preliminary studies. Other supplements include SAM-e, known for relieving pain, and *Boswellia serrate* (also called Indian frankincense).

Rheumatoid Arthritis

Rheumatoid arthritis (RA) is practically a different disease than osteoarthritis. It's character-ized by inflamed knuckles and joints and, often, misshapen hands. People who have RA and other forms of arthritis must endure endless episodes of swollen, red, painfully stiff joints.

RA, like the related disorder lupus, is an autoimmune disease, which means the body is lit-erally attacking itself. And the battle isn't confined to the joints. The entire body is affected, sometimes causing fatigue, loss of appetite, even fever.

The desperation bred by the mystery and misery of RA could explain why, according to esti-mates, most sufferers have tried as many as 13 different arthritis remedies in search of relief. Diets and food cures seem to lead the pack. In addition to diet, some relief from discomfort may also be found through weight loss and exercise. Tai chi is particularly recommended. Hot and cold packs may help control pain, as may massage.

NSAIDs, steroids, and DMARDs (disease-modifying antirheumatic drugs) may also be pre-scribed. A combination of DMARDs and a newer class of drugs called biologics may, in fact, be able to produce remission.

Surgery may also be an option: from joint fusion to a total joint replacement.

Other supplements that are commonly recommended include thunder god vine, which unfortunately causes side effects that include stomach upset, headache, and even sterility; topical creams that include cap-saicin; an anti-inflammatory called cat's claw; and gamma linolenic acids, or GLA. Before taking a sup-plement, you should always consider the potential side effects and check with your doctor on potential interactions with medications you're taking.

gamma-linolenic acid

Foods to Eat and Avoid

The Arthritis Foundation recommends that people diagnosed with RA eat anti-inflammatory foods. There's evidence that the Mediterranean diet—low on meat, high on fish, vegetables, and olive oil—provides a wide array of health benefits, including fighting inflammatory condi-tions. The omega-3 fatty acids in fatty fish such as salmon, tuna, and sardines are especially beneficial, and your doctor may point you towards a fish oil supplement in addition to encour-aging you to eat fish regularly. Nuts and berries are also inflammation fighters.

Processed foods can increase inflammation. In general, foods like sugar, saturated fats, and high levels of salt that are known for impairing heart health are also foods to avoid if you want to decrease inflammation levels.

The Arthritis Foundation recommends incorporating a number of anti-inflammatory spices in your cooking: garlic, ginger, cinnamon, cayenne—and turmeric. Black pepper may help your body better absorb the turmeric.

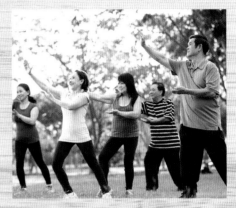

Exercise such as tai chi may help reduce pain and increase mobility.

Turmeric and Osteoarthritis

Several studies have been conducted on the use of turmeric or curcumin supplements to treat the pain of osteoarthritis. For example, a 2009 study based in Thailand focused on 107 patients with osteoarthritis in the knee. The study concluded that *Curcuma domestica* extracts were comparable to ibuprofen in how well they treated pain. Two studies published in 2014, which also focused on patients with knee osteoarthritis and compared pain reduction when patients were given a form of curcumin/curcuminoids vs. a placebo, also showed positive results. Note that studies have focused on extracts and supplements, which involve higher dosages of turmeric than would be accessed through food, not just simply incorporating turmeric in your diet. A meta-analytic review of those studies and several others concluded that while results were promising, larger studies were needed.

Turmeric and Rheumatoid Arthritis

Small research studies on the use of curcumin have shown positive results for preventing joint inflammation, reducing joint inflammation, and alleviating pain associated with rheumatoid arthritis. For instance, one small 2012 study divided patients into three groups. One group took 500 milligrams of curcumin, another took 50 milligrams of diclofenac sodium, and a third took both. All three groups benefited from treatment. Not only was pain reduced, but tenderness of joints was as well. Curcumin, however, produced the superior result in that study, and it did so without side effects. (While side effects such as digestive upset can occur with high dosages, they would usually not occur at normal dosages.) Further studies are needed before definitive conclusions can be drawn, however. And while turmeric may successfully treat symptoms of RA, it is not claimed to bring about remission in the same way that DMARDs and biologics can—in other words, while turmeric may be one helpful tool in your treatment plan for RA, it wouldn't replace medication altogether.

Aging

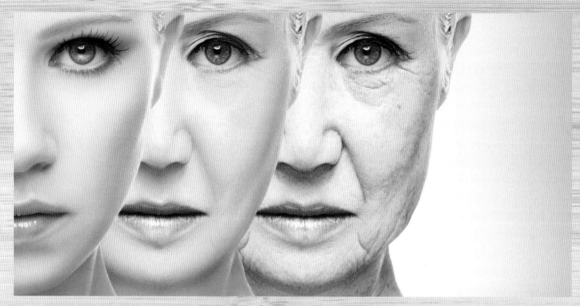

Aging is an inevitable part of life. And while some people embrace "aging gracefully," many of us prefer to seek out ways to make the clock tick just a bit slower. Lucky for us, turmeric may be one of best weapons we have in our anti-aging arsenal.

What Causes Aging?

Cells, the most basic body unit, are at the center of any discussion about aging. You have trillions of cells, and they're organized into different tissues that make up organs, such as your brain, heart, and skin.

Some cells, such as those that line the gastrointestinal tract, reproduce continuously; others, such as the cells on the inside of arteries, lie dormant but are capable of replicating in response to injury. Still others, including cells of the heart, nerves, and muscles, cannot reproduce. Some of these non-reproducing cells have short life spans and must be continually replaced by other cells in the body. (Red and white blood cells are examples.) Others, such as heart and nerve cells, live for years or even decades.

Over time, cell death outpaces cell production, leaving us with fewer cells. As a result, we are less capable of repairing wear and tear on the body, and our immune system is compromised. We become more susceptible to infections and less proficient at seeking out and destroying mutant cells that could cause cancerous tumors. In fact, many older adults succumb to conditions they could have resisted in their youth.

Genes or Lifestyle?

Genes are powerful predictors of health and longevity as well as disease and death, but they're only part of the story. If your parents and grandparents lived well into their nineties, chances are you will, too—but not if you abuse your body along the way. While genes partially determine who will develop chronic conditions that hasten the aging process, such as cancer and heart disease, there is no question that a healthy lifestyle is your weapon against the genes you've been dealt, or your ace in the hole if you've got good genes.

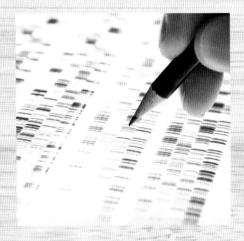

Healthy living delays many of the body changes that aging brings. And it's never too late to start on the road to better health. Eating a nutritious diet goes a long way toward insuring good health. For instance, getting enough calcium and vitamin D at any age will retard the onset, and the progression, of osteoporosis, a bone disease that causes pain, fractures, hospitalization, and even death in the elderly. If you're a smoker and you quit at any time, you decrease the chances of having a heart attack. And exercising or becoming more physically active improves lung function and lowers the risk for heart attack, no matter how old you are.

Turmeric

Physical age is only one of the factors that contributes to the wrinkles, sagging skin, and age spots that develop as we get older. Other influences include pollution, eating habits, and sun exposure. All of these eventually result in a loss of collagen and elastin, proteins that help keep skin firm and young-looking. But research has shown that turmeric inhibits an enzyme called elastase, which prevents elastin from forming, by up to 65 percent. And turmeric's antioxidants help to counter the effects of oxidative stress, which can result in premature signs of aging.

Ingesting around a teaspoon of turmeric a day is a good way to get the anti-aging, antioxidant benefits of the spice, but it can also be used topically in your skin care routine. Try mixing a teaspoon of turmeric with a teaspoon of honey and a bit of coconut oil to make a face mask, or look for skin care products containing turmeric at your favorite store.

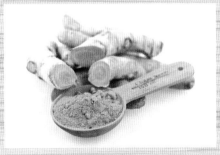

Alzheimer's Disease

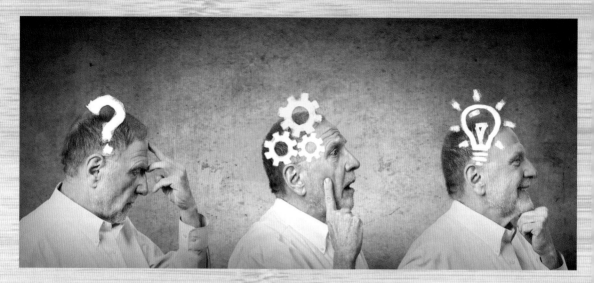

Alzheimer's disease (AD) is many people's worst nightmare. Most diseases destroy either a physical or a mental function. Alzheimer's seizes both, slowly and steadily destroying memory, logical thought, and language. Simple tasks—how to eat or comb hair—are forgotten, and once AD sets in there's no turning back the clock.

The disease is named for Dr. Alois Alzheimer, a German doctor who, during an autopsy in 1906, discovered physical changes in the brain of a woman who had died of a strange mental illness. He found plaques and tangles in her brain, signs that are now considered hallmarks of AD.

A Progressive Disease

AD is one of a group of brain disorders called dementia, which are progressive degenerative brain syndromes that affect memory, thinking, behavior, and emotion. Alzheimer's is the most common cause of dementia: Between 50 and 60 percent of all cases of dementia can be attributed to Alzheimer's.

Early symptoms include difficulty remembering names, places, or faces and trouble recalling things that just happened. Personality changes and confusion when driving a car or handling money are also early symptoms. Eventually mild forgetfulness progresses to problems in comprehension, speaking, reading, and writing. And physical breakdown occurs, too, partly because tasks such as eating and drinking are simply forgotten or too difficult to accomplish. Unfortunately, there is no cure for Alzheimer's, although some medications may help manage symptoms.

Kitchen Tips for Caregivers

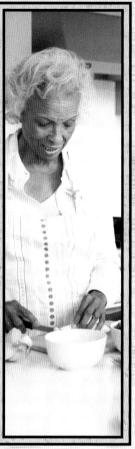

- Using utensils can become difficult for people with Alzheimer's, so solve the problem by offering finger foods. Keep them simple, handy, and nutritious.

- Almonds are rich in vitamin E, which may delay the progression of AD. Two ounces of almonds a day supplies the recommended amount of vitamin E.

- One of the most common problems plaguing people with AD is low fluid intake. Those with the disease simply forget to drink, or they choose not to in order to avoid bathroom emergencies and accidents. The result is dehydration, which can cause a loss of potassium, which in turn, contributes to confusion. The simple solution for restoring essential potassium to the body is to force fluids—water or sports drinks with potassium—but that's often easier said than done. Bananas are a great option, both a source of fast energy and easy to chew and swallow.

- Don't serve foods with pits or bones.

- Always check food temperature. Hot and cold sensations can be numbed in people with AD, but they still can get burned.

- Don't serve foods with a mixture of textures. They may be hard to swallow.

- Serve foods that require little chewing, such as soups, ground meat, and applesauce.

- Serve several smaller meals instead of three main meals.

- Select favorite foods, especially if the appetite is poor. And keep in mind that as the disease progresses, food preferences may change.

- Play music at meals. Mealtimes can be stressful and music is relaxing. Choose songs from the patient's youth or that hold a special memory.

Turmeric

As one of the cruelest diseases associated with aging, Alzheimer's is often studied in the hopes that a cure will be found. Recently, there has been much research on the effect of turmeric on the disease, and the findings have been quite promising. While there is little evidence that the spice itself can be used to treat the disorder, some of the compounds contained within it are showing fascinating results.

First, in lab studies, curcumin has been shown to break up amyloid-beta plaques, which form in the brains of those with Alzheimer's disease. It is possible that curcumin could one day be the key to targeting these areas of the brain. Second, scientists are also studying a compound in turmeric called turmerone, which can stimulate stem cells to create new brain cells. Although this research is very new, finding a way to create new brain cells would be life-changing for those with Alzheimer's and dementia. While anecdotal evidence, such as the low rates of Alzheimer's disease in India, suggests turmeric may be helpful at preventing the disorder, the scientific evidence surrounding the golden spice may ultimately prove to be groundbreaking.

Depression

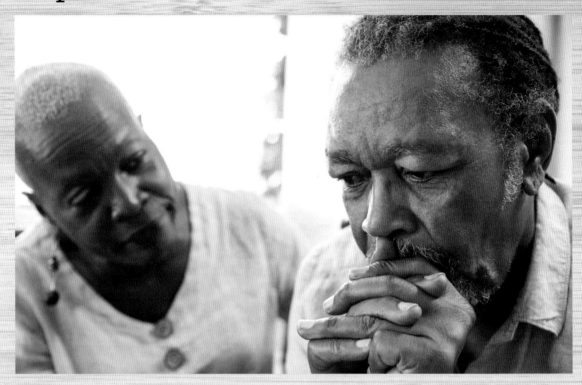

We all feel sad or stressed out now and then; the struggles of life make sure of it! But for some individuals, those moods begin to feel overwhelming and last for weeks or months at a time, preventing them from living life to the fullest.

Symptoms

Depression is characterized by several symptoms, including a depressive mood, lack of energy, feelings of worthlessness, lack of focus, and sleeping disorders. People who suffer with the condition can also be irritable, eat too much (or not enough), feel anxious, or even have physical symptoms like headaches, joint pain, or digestive trouble. And depression can make other physical issues—especially chronic pain—feel even worse.

The disorder can affect anyone, although women are twice as likely as men to be depressed. And experts believe genetics play a role: If you have a parent who has struggled with depression, you are more likely to experience it. The cause of the disorder is still unknown, but doctors believe it may be connected to altered brain chemistry. Communication between brain cells that regulate mood may work less efficiently in those with depression, causing an imbalance of the neurotransmitters serotonin, norepinephrine, and dopamine.

Traditional Treatment for Depression

With mild to moderate depression, talk therapy can often help, as it aims to change thoughts and behaviors that contribute to the feelings, or helps sufferers work through issues with relationships or unresolved issues. Exercise can also be a great way to help stave off mild depression, as it increases mood-boosting endorphins, plus helps increase energy and improve sleep. Other depression-busters include maintaining a supportive social circle (whether that be friends and family, support groups, or taking classes at a gym), or even adopting a pet—studies have shown that pet owners have better overall health than those who don't have a furry friend.

But for those who don't find relief through these channels, medications may be prescribed that help to balance the neurotransmitters in the brain. These antidepressants may take several weeks to take effect, and can come with many unpleasant side effects, such as nausea, weight gain, fatigue, irritability, or constipation. Worse yet, antidepressants may eventually stop working for some people, leading to more medications, and in younger people, antidepressants can actually increase suicidal thoughts and behavior.

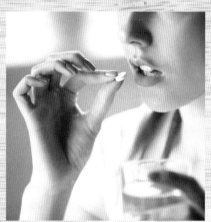

Turmeric

The effects of turmeric on depression have been well-studied and documented. There is mounting evidence that the spice not only helps to relieve symptoms of depression, but it also may work just as well as prescription antidepressants. This could be huge news for those who suffer from depression, but who also suffer side effects from conventional medications.

It is believed that inflammation can lead to changes in the brain that interfere with the production of the neurotransmitters serotonin and dopamine, which help to regulate mood. The anti-inflammatory properties of turmeric help to bring balance back to these hormones, and strengthen the brain's ability to regulate them. One major study even showed that curcumin alone works almost as well as Prozac in relieving symptoms of depression, and when combined with an antidepressant, it increases the efficacy of the medication.

One day, turmeric may be commonly prescribed for depression, but in the meantime, supplements—or even a daily turmeric latte—may be helpful. A word of caution: if you already take antidepressants, be sure to ask your doctor before adding turmeric or switching to supplements altogether.

High Cholesterol

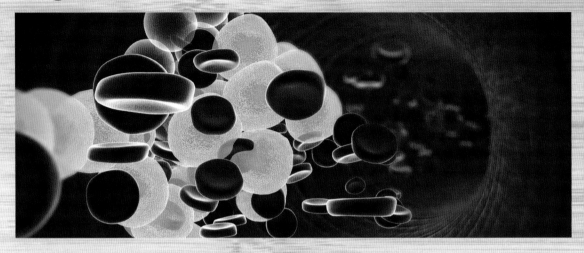

Cholesterol is that waxy, soft stuff that floats around in your bloodstream as well as in all the cells in your body. It takes a bad rap these days because the word cholesterol strikes fear in the hearts of even the healthiest of people. Having cholesterol in your blood is normal and even healthy because it's used in the formation of cell membranes, tissues, and essential hormones. So, in proper amounts, cholesterol is good. In excessive amounts, though, it can clog the arteries leading to your heart and cause coronary disease, heart attack, or stroke.

How Cholesterol Builds Up

Cholesterol comes from two sources: the foods you eat and your very own liver. And the truth of the matter is, your liver can produce all the cholesterol your body will ever need. This means that what you get in your food isn't necessary. Some people get rid of extra cholesterol easily through normal bodily waste mechanisms, but others hang on to it because their bodies just aren't as efficient in removing it, which puts them at risk.

So, what makes people prone to high blood cholesterol?

- Family history
- Eating too many foods high in saturated fats
- Diabetes
- Kidney and liver disorders
- Alcoholism
- Obesity
- Smoking
- Stress

Good and Bad Cholesterol?

There are two different kinds of cholesterol, and yes, one's good and one's bad. Cholesterol can't get around on its own, so it hitches a ride from lipoproteins to get to the body's cells. Problem is, there are two different rigs picking it up: One is called HDL, or high-density lipoprotein, the other is called LDL, or low-density lipoprotein. HDL is the good ride; it travels away from your arteries. LDL is the bad ride; it heads straight to your arteries. Bottom line: HDL is what you want more of; you want less of LDL.

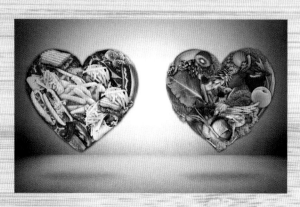

Traditional Treatment

High cholesterol can be cured two ways: by medication and/or by diet. There are numerous effective drugs on the market that will make drastic reductions in cholesterol levels, but they all come with side effects and require frequent blood tests to monitor for possible problems. But there are alternative cures, and they may work on their own or along with conventional treatment. Whatever your cure, it must come with advice from your doctor since your heart is at risk.

Turmeric

Keeping cholesterol low—especially low-density lipoprotein, or LDL, cholesterol—is important for overall heart health. Fortunately, recent studies have shown that turmeric may help to lower not only LDL cholesterol, but triglycerides (a type of fat also associated with heart disease) as well. Studies have shown that curcumin is able to prevent cholesterol production in the liver and to block the absorption of cholesterol in the digestive system. It has also been shown to prevent the formation of oxidized LDL, an especially harmful type of cholesterol that contributes to a hardening of the arteries. One promising study suggested that curcumin can help lower oxidized LDL by around 30 percent, and lower overall cholesterol by almost 12 percent. Research has also demonstrated that one gram of curcumin a day can lower triglycerides after only 30 days. The effects of turmeric on cholesterol are still being studied, so as of yet there is no recommended amount to consume. But experts agree that adding more turmeric to your diet is a heart-healthy way to help keep cholesterol in check.

Heart Health

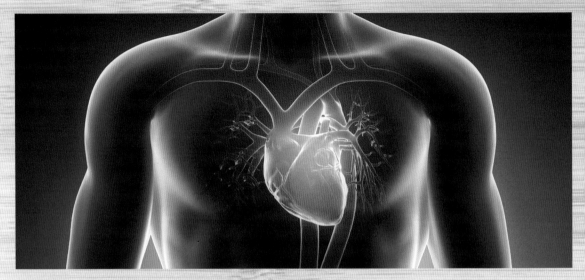

The heart is an amazing structure, tough yet fragile. A muscle, its network of arteries and veins transport blood through your body, nourishing organs and tissues. When the heart is working as it should, you barely notice it. But when your heart starts acting strangely, you have cause to worry. Thankfully, we live in a day when heart disease can be treated very successfully, and in some cases, the condition can even be reversed.

Heart Trouble

Heart disease is any condition that keeps your heart from functioning at its best or causes a deterioration of the heart's arteries and vessels. Coronary heart disease (CHD), also known as coronary artery disease, is the most common form of heart disease, affecting millions of people in America. If you are diagnosed with CHD, it means you have atherosclerosis, or hardening of the arteries on the heart's surface. Arteries become hard when plaque accumulates on artery walls.

This plaque develops gradually as an overabundance of low-density lipoprotein (LDL) cholesterol (the bad stuff) makes itself at home in your arteries. The plaque builds and narrows the artery walls, making it more and more difficult for blood to pass through the heart and increasing the opportunity for a blood clot to form. If the heart doesn't get enough blood, it can cause chest pain (angina) or a heart attack. Not treating coronary heart disease can also lead to congestive heart failure (CHF). CHF happens when your heart isn't strong enough to pump blood throughout the body—it fails to meet the body's need for oxygen. This often causes congestion in the lungs and a variety of other problems for your heart and the rest of your body.

Honing In on Heart Disease

There are many risk factors for heart disease, some you can do something about, and some you can't. A family history of heart disease puts you at much greater risk for developing it yourself. While you can't do anything about your genes, there are a number of risk factors that you can control. These are the ones you can do something about:

- High levels of low-density lipoprotein (LDL) cholesterol (the bad stuff), and low levels of high-density lipoprotein (the good stuff).
- High levels of triglycerides. Triglyceride levels increase when you eat too many fatty foods or when you eat too much—excess calories are made into triglycerides and stored as fat in cells. Having an abundance of triglycerides has been linked to coronary heart disease.
- High blood pressure
- Smoking
- Lack of regular exercise
- A high fat diet
- Being overweight or obese
- Diabetes
- Ongoing stress or depression

Turmeric

Aspirin has long been used as a preventive measure to help prevent heart attacks, by reducing the body's blood clotting abilities. This is especially important if blood vessels are already narrowed by fatty deposits—a potential blood clot can easily block blood flow to the heart. But turmeric may provide the same blood-thinning protection as aspirin, in a more natural, gentle way, because it acts as an antiplatelet agent that can slow the formation of blood clots.

This action has been especially well documented in heart surgery patients. Clinical research has shown that bypass patients who take four grams of curcumin daily beginning three days prior to surgery and continuing for five days post-surgery reduce their risk of surgery-related heart attack by up to 65 percent.

Turmeric has also been shown to improve the function of the endothelium, which are the cells that line the interior of blood vessels. Dysfunctional endothelium cells can lead to a condition known as nonobstructive coronary artery disease, which causes chronic chest pain and can lead to high blood pressure and other issues.

Of course, turmeric should not be seen as a replacement for exercise and a healthy diet, but there's no doubt the spice makes a great addition to a healthy lifestyle.

Diabetes

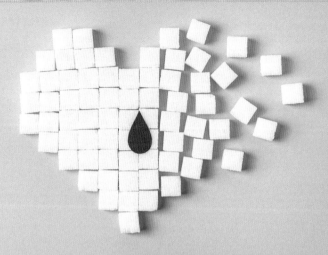

Diabetes is now the seventh leading cause of death in the United States. With more than 100 million Americans living with diabetes or prediabetes—a condition that can lead to type 2 diabetes if not treated—treatment and prevention of this disease is more important than ever. And research is showing that turmeric might be able to help.

What Is Diabetes?

Diabetes is a disease that reduces, or stops, the body's ability to produce or respond to insulin, a hormone produced in the pancreas. Insulin's role is to open the door for glucose, a form of sugar, to enter the body's cells so that it can be used for energy. When the body has a problem metabolizing glucose, it builds up in the blood, and the body's cells starve. There are two major types of diabetes:

Type 1. The body produces no insulin at all, and daily insulin shots are required. This disease used to be called juvenile diabetes because there is a higher rate of diagnosis among children ages 10 to 14. It is also referred to as insulin-dependent diabetes because injections of insulin are required to control blood glucose. The cause isn't known, but Type 1 tends to run in families. A much smaller number of people with diabetes have Type 1—only five percent.

Type 2. This is the most common form of diabetes, and it occurs when the body is insulin resistant. That could be either because the body fails to make enough insulin or because it doesn't properly use the insulin it does produce. The cause is often poor dietary habits, sedentary lifestyle, and obesity. Those with Type 2 may or may not need oral medication or insulin, depending on how their body responds to changes in diet and exercise.

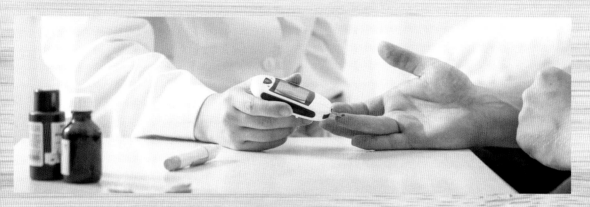

Blood Sugar Control

There is no cure for diabetes, but it can be controlled. And control is essential because diabetes can lead to heart disease, stroke, kidney disease and failure, blindness, and amputation if not treated. Fortunately, diet, exercise, and stress reduction can play a huge part in managing symptoms and stalling the progression of the disease. Medications, and eventually insulin, can also help. Knowledge is key for those affected by diabetes, who need to check their blood sugar level frequently.

A simple blood test called hemoglobin A1C (also called HbA1C) can measure your cumulative average blood sugar levels for the past three months. It's the best test to find out whether your blood sugar is under control. People with diabetes should have a hemoglobin A1C test at least every six months. The goal is a finding of 7 percent. That's because a major diabetes study shows that those whose results were 7 percent or lower had a much better chance of delaying or preventing diabetes complications related to the eyes, kidneys, and nerves than those whose levels were 8 percent or higher.

Turmeric

Studies have found that curcumin has numerous beneficial effects on those with diabetes, including reducing the production of glucose and glycogen in the liver, improving cell function in the pancreas, stimulating insulin production, and reducing insulin resistance. Even more promising, a study that was published in the American Diabetic Association's journal, *Diabetes Care*, found that 250 milligrams of curcumin taken six times a day for nine months prevented the development of type 2 diabetes in 100 percent of prediabetics.

These findings are especially encouraging to patients who take medication to control diabetes, some of which can cause side effects, vitamin deficiencies, and even increase the risk of strokes. Research has even shown that curcumin may be more effective than metformin, one of the most commonly prescribed medications for diabetes.

Cancer and Cancer Treatment

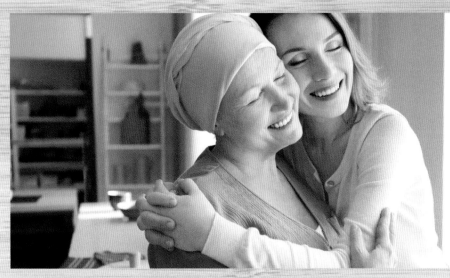

Cancer isn't a single disease. Cancer is an umbrella term for more than 200 different conditions, which all have in common the out-of-control growth of cells. Each type of cancer is unique, with its own set of triggers and treatments.

Cancer and Your Diet

Proving a dietary link to cancer is not easy. Although the connection to some types of cancer seems more solid, some suspected ties are merely educated guesses based on statistics from epidemiology. Epidemiology is a branch of science that observes and compares the rates of diseases in different environments and situations. Actual clinical trials that put theories to the ultimate test are expensive and difficult to design, and they cannot provide valid results for decades, because cancer takes that long to develop. For years, scientists focused on specific substances in foods that might cause cancer. At first, suspicions centered around manmade creations, such as additives, artificial sweeteners, and pesticides. Then researchers refocused their attention on the many natural toxins in foods that were potentially cancerous, such as aflatoxins in peanuts and solanine in potatoes. Today, the dietary fight against cancer has progressed further still. These days, when we talk about taking dietary steps to prevent cancer, we're talking about being proactive. Today's preventive strategies go beyond simply avoiding potentially cancer-causing substances in certain foods to actually using diet to strengthen the body's defenses against cancer and toxic substances. Indeed, there's more and more evidence that what you do eat can actually offer protection against, and therefore lower your chances of developing, cancer. Food has gone from enemy to ally. What's more, a diet that may help protect against cancer appears remarkably similar to a diet that is heart healthy and weight wise as well.

Anti-cancer Crusaders

Just think fruits and vegetables. Study after study has linked a low incidence of cancer with eating lots of fruits and veggies. And it's no wonder. Fruits and vegetables pack in both types of fiber—soluble and insoluble. They are virtually devoid of fat, as long as you can resist adding butter, margarine, cheese, or high-fat sauces and salad dressings. And fresh produce is your best bet for getting plenty of vitamin C and beta-carotene—two important antioxidant nutrients. And, lastly, fruits and vegetables boast a wide array of mysterious and promising cancer-fighting phytochemicals, such as sulforaphane in broccoli, indoles in cabbage, and liminoids in citrus fruits. In short, they're just what the epidemiologist ordered.

Foods to Avoid

While you're opting for more foods with cancer-fighting properties, you should also keep tabs on your intake of certain foods and other aspects of your overall diet that may actually aid cancer's growth or development and do your best to limit these. Adding potentially helpful foods and losing possible dietary dangers can equal a more cancer-protective diet all around.

Fat has been found guilty in contributing to the development of a number of diseases, and cancer is no exception. High-fat diets have been linked to an increase in the risk of cancers of the colon, rectum, prostate, and endometrium.

There's also no doubt that alcohol contributes to esophageal and oral-cavity cancers. Add cigarette smoke, and the risk skyrockets. There have been conflicting data on moderate drinking and breast-cancer risk. It's probably best to follow the advice given for other chronic diseases: If you drink, do so only in moderation.

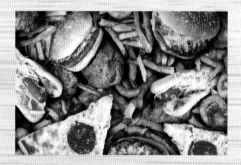

Mutagens are substances that can set off sudden changes in a cell's genetic makeup, creating potentially cancerous compounds. Whenever you brown food, mutagens may form. The more well-done your meat is, the more mutagens you are likely to consume. Because these mutagens don't form until meat is at 300 degrees Fahrenheit for a significant time, rare or medium-rare meat is not affected. Microwaving, boiling, and baking are safer methods of cooking than grilling and broiling because the cooking temperatures are typically lower, so use these methods more often than the higher-temperature methods.

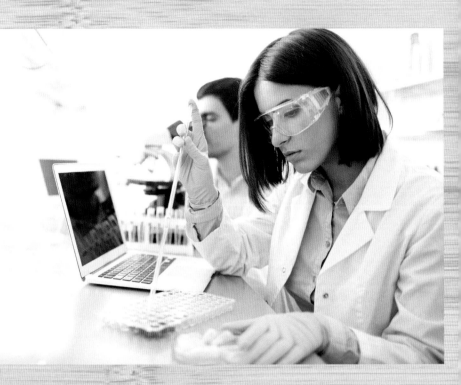

Turmeric and Cancer

Cancer is such an insidious disease that it's hard to believe a natural remedy could affect it in any way. But turmeric is showing so much promise in laboratory studies as a way to prevent and treat cancer, that even big names in research, including the Mayo Clinic and Memorial Sloan Kettering Cancer Center, are taking notice.

Curcumin has displayed protective effects against colon, stomach, and skin cancers in laboratory tests, and has been shown to stop the replication of tumor cells when directly applied to them. It has also proven to be biologically active in patients with pancreatic cancer, leading researchers to continue studying its possible use as a future cancer treatment.

In addition, there is evidence that curcumin may make chemotherapy more effective and may protect healthy cells from damage during radiation therapy. But the spice can also interfere with certain chemotherapy drugs, so more study is needed to understand its possible role in cancer treatment.

Although most research concerning cancer and turmeric has been lab-based and conducted on animals, human studies have begun and will hopefully yield some encouraging results.

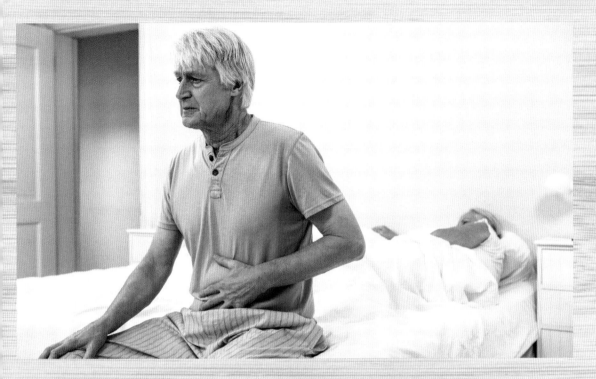

Turmeric and Cancer Side Effects

As if a cancer diagnosis isn't stressful enough, oftentimes patients must endure months of painful and uncomfortable side effects while undergoing treatments. Finding ways to lessen these symptoms is vitally important for maintaining a positive attitude and living as normal a life as possible. But many cancer patients are wary about adding another pharmaceutical drug into their daily rotation of medications, and instead search for natural remedies. Recent research is discovering that turmeric may be just the solution many are looking for.

One of the most common side effects of chemotherapy is gastrointestinal toxicity, which results in vomiting, diarrhea, and nausea. But research has shown that curcumin has a protective effect on the gastrointestinal tract, and if taken 24 hours prior to starting chemotherapy, greatly reduces these unpleasant symptoms. Curcumin has also been shown to protect other healthy cells from chemotherapy-induced damage, preventing side effects such as liver or kidney damage, nerve pain, and decreased immunity.

While the golden spice may be an excellent choice to help ensure a healthy, happy quality of life while undergoing cancer treatment, it's important to note that turmeric may interfere with certain chemotherapy drugs, so be sure to consult your doctor before taking any supplements.

Digestive Issues

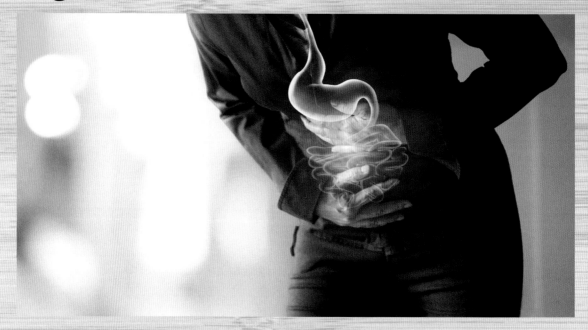

We all deal with digestion issues now and then. Whether it be heartburn, nausea, gas, or diarrhea, the symptoms can be unpleasant, painful, and disruptive, prompting a search for the best remedy. Fortunately, we may need to look no further than our spice rack.

How Digestion Works

When you eat something, the digestive process begins right away in your mouth. Your salivary glands produce digestive juices that lubricate your food and prepare fat for digestion. The food travels through your esophagus into your stomach, where digestive juices continue to break food down even further so it can travel on to the small intestine. The pancreas and liver secrete other digestive juices that flow into the small intestines. In the small intestine, vital nutrients including vitamins, minerals, water, salt, carbohydrates, and proteins are sucked out of the food and absorbed into your body. By the time your dinner makes its way to the large intestines, it's mostly bulk and water. The large intestines absorb the water and help you get rid of the excess.

When Things Go Awry

But sometimes things in the digestive system go awry and cause indigestion, a catchall term that means you simply have trouble digesting your food. When you eat too much, or you eat the wrong foods, you may get one of a number of indigestion symptoms: nausea, vomiting, heartburn, bloating, or gas.

Those unpleasant feelings may send you running to the drugstore for relief, and if they do, you've got plenty of company. The American Gastroenterological Association says that digestive problems are one of the most common reasons Americans take over-the-counter medications. Indigestion can be a symptom of something more serious, such as gastritis, an ulcer, severe heartburn, irritable bowel syndrome, or diverticulitis.

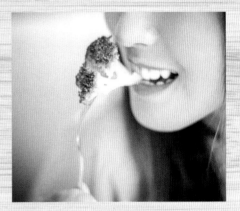

Some people get relief for occasional bouts of digestive woes through lifestyle remedies: cutting coffee and alcohol, which may irritate the system, as well as common culprit foods such as pepper, broccoli, cabbage, and Brussels sprouts. Eating slowly can help, as can eating smaller meals spaced throughout the day. This keeps you from overloading your stomach all at once but also ensures that your stomach isn't empty, allowing acid to build up. Apples have enough fiber to help reset your digestive system.

Away from the kitchen table, regular exercise is a good way to help your digestive system stay healthy—aside from other benefits, exercise also helps lower high stress levels, which can wreak havoc on a person's digestive system.

Folk Remedies

A number of herbs and spices have historically been used to counter indigestion: cardamom, caraway seeds, cinnamon, fennel seeds, ginger, mint, catnip, chamomile, and thyme among them. Mint should not be used for heartburn, though, as it can help the stomach muscle to relax, letting acids into the esophagus.

Turmeric

Turmeric has been shown to relieve a host of digestive issues. For instance, studies show that consuming a teaspoon of the spice twice a day can improve the function of the esophagus and colon, as well as preventing acid and bile overproduction that can lead to indigestion and nausea. The anti-inflammatory compounds in turmeric help to relieve stomach pain from overeating or indulging in fatty or spicy foods.

Magnesium and potassium in the spice help to keep fluids balanced for those suffering with diarrhea. A teaspoon taken up to three times a day can be a welcome remedy for this condition. And to treat symptoms of gas, experts recommend stirring a tablespoon of turmeric into an eight-ounce glass of juice and sipping the concoction to prevent the overproduction of acids that cause gas.

Inflammatory Bowel Diseases

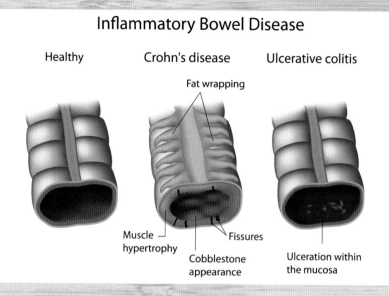

Inflammatory Bowel Disease

Some 1.6 million Americans suffer from inflammatory bowel diseases, which includes disorders like ulcerative colitis and Crohn's disease. They can be an extremely disruptive and debilitating issue that causes an impaired quality of life. Many patients need to take drugs every day, which may help to control symptoms but can also cause side effects like vomiting, headaches, rashes, and inflammation of the kidneys, liver, or pancreas. Inflammatory bowel disease should not be confused with inflammatory bowel syndrome, a disorder affecting muscle contractions of the colon and not linked to an inflammation of the intestines, as are Crohn's and colitis.

Ulcerative Colitis

Ulcerative colitis is a chronic disease of the large intestine, also known as the colon, in which the lining of the colon becomes inflamed and develops tiny open sores, or ulcers, that produce pus and mucous. The combination of inflammation and ulceration can cause abdominal discomfort and frequent emptying of the colon.

Ulcerative colitis is the result of an abnormal response by your body's immune system. Crohn's disease can affect any part of the gastrointestinal tract, but ulcerative colitis affects only the colon. Additionally, while Crohn's disease can affect all layers of the bowel wall, ulcerative colitis only affects the colon's lining. Half of patients with ulcerative colitis experience mild to severe symptoms, including constant diarrhea, abdominal pain, blood in the stool, as well as loss of appetite, weight loss and fatigue. The symptoms can come and go often with months, if not longer, of remission.

Colitis Treatments

Medication to reduce inflammation is one of many ways to lessen the symptoms of colitis. Patients are also given dietary and lifestyle suggestions to keep the disease at bay, and often are restricted from eating dairy products. In about one-fourth to one-third of the patients, surgery may also be an option. The surgery may involve removing the colon and rectum and inserting a device in the skin from which wastes get emptied. Newer surgeries today often can be done without having to insert a device into the skin.

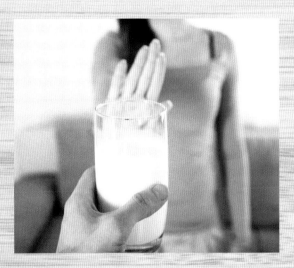

Crohn's Disease

Treatment for this disease can often include many different medications, such as anti-inflammatory drugs, corticosteroids, immune system modifiers, antibiotics, and nutritional supplements. Surgery is an unfortunate necessity for up to seventy-five percent of Crohn's patients, and can consist of removing the diseased parts of the intestines and joining healthy ends together. While this surgery can help people remain symptom-free for years, it does not cure the disease, and Crohn's may eventually return.

Turmeric

Recent research has studied the effects of turmeric on those with inflammatory bowel disease, and the results have been extremely promising. In one study, a group of IBD sufferers in remission were given curcumin in addition to their usual medications, and another was given a placebo. The group taking curcumin only had a 5 percent rate of relapse, compared to a 20 percent rate of relapse in the placebo group. What's more, when the curcumin group stopped taking the supplement, their rate of relapse rose to the same rate as the placebo group.

Curcumin also caused zero side effects in the study participants. Although more research needs to be done, including exploring curcumin's effects aside from other medications, it seems that curcumin may one day prove to be a much more gentle and natural remedy for those struggling with inflammatory bowel diseases.

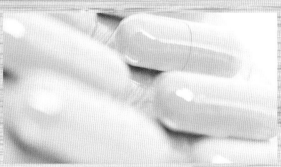

Skin Problems

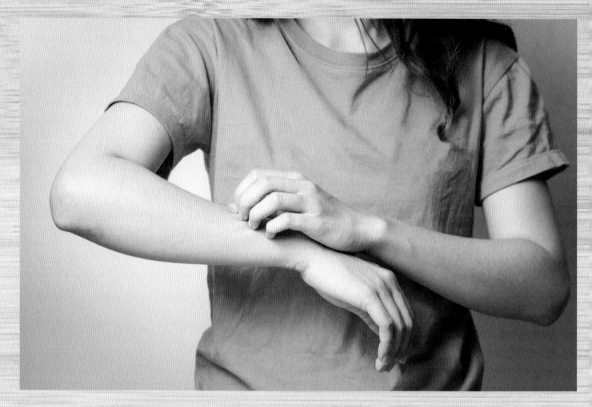

The largest organ in our bodies is the skin. It serves us well by absorbing oxygen as well as nutrients such as Vitamin D. Hormonal imbalances, diet, disrupted immune system, and allergies can all cause skin problems. Our skin is deluged by a host of enemies including cold, windy weather, insect bites, heat, and overexposure to allergies and the sun, as well as a stressed immune system. These can cause dry, itchy skin, rashes, sores, burns, and discoloration. And, of course, in the case of sunburn, there's the possibility of skin cancer. Various creams, sprays, and other products are prescribed to help reduce these symptoms.

Folk Remedies

There have also been any number of folk and natural remedies used throughout the years to settle skin problems. Chamomile tea, oatmeal in bathwater, milk, and aloe vera have all been used to treat sunburn. A paste of almonds and honey have been used as a gentle facial scrub suitable for oily skin. For those with dry skin, oatmeal can soothe it, and salt after a shower or bath can help leave skin smooth. A bath of basil tea can be used to treat hives—and oatmeal in bathwater shows up once again as a remedy to ease the itches caused by hives.

Turmeric & Healing Spices

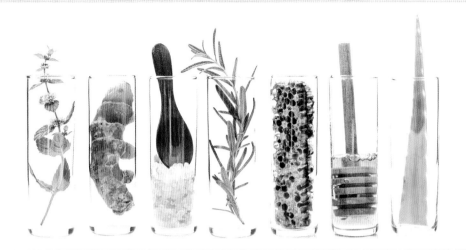

Turmeric

One Google search is all you need to see the variety of skincare products on the market that contain turmeric. Everything from creams to serums to masks can be purchased from vendors by skincare-savvy shoppers. And it's no wonder: The anti-inflammatory and antioxidant properties of turmeric give it a host of complexion-friendly benefits.

In fact, turmeric is so prized for its skincare abilities in India that the spice is applied to the skin of a bride and groom before their wedding during a *haldi* ceremony, in order to give the skin a glow. But the spice does more than give brides and grooms a youthful glow. It also helps to calm redness due to acne, eczema, and rosacea, and can prevent new blemishes from forming.

There are plenty of turmeric lotions and potions to choose from at drugstores and online, but it's easy to mix up your own skin-soothing salve. Experts recommend applying a mixture of honey and turmeric to affected areas to calm skin. Leave the turmeric/honey blend on your skin for about 20 minutes, then rinse with cool water.

You can make a simple acne gel by adding one part turmeric to two parts honey, and using it to spot treat blemishes. Or mix up a paste of aloe vera gel and turmeric, and use it to calm the itch from bug bites, poison ivy, or eczema.

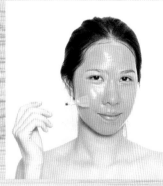

Turmeric is also known to improve circulation, which can help reduce undereye puffiness and lighten dark circles. And the spice helps to protect against fine lines, age spots, and dryness due to sun damage, whether applied topically or ingested.

Hay Fever

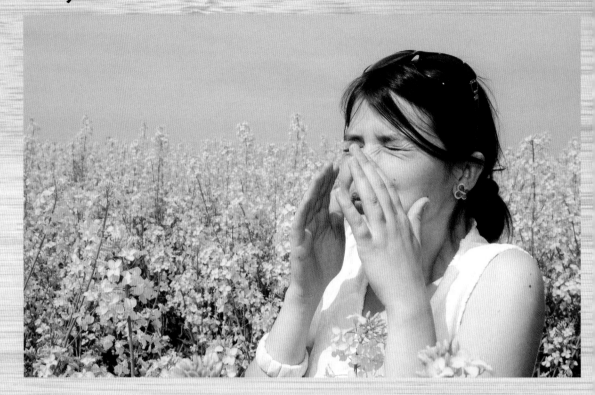

Seasonal allergies can be miserable, bringing with them bouts of sneezing, itchy eyes, and a runny nose. And although there are many over-the-counter and prescription medications to help keep symptoms at bay, these often come with side effects like drowsiness and dry mouth. Many allergy sufferers have begun searching for natural remedies for their sneezing and itching, and turmeric may be exactly what they're looking for.

When your body encounters an allergen, such as ragweed or pollen, the immune system reacts as if the substance is a harmful foreign invader and creates histamines. The histamines try to rid the body of this "harmful" substance, causing the familiar symptoms of seasonal allergies.

How Allergies Work

Normally, the immune system guards against intruders it considers harmful to the body, such as certain viruses and bacteria. That's its job. However, in allergic people, the immune system goes a bit bonkers. It overreacts when you breathe, ingest, or touch a harmless substance. The benign culprits triggering the overreaction, such as dust, pet dander, and pollen, are called allergens.

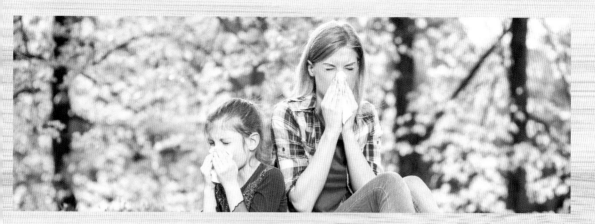

The body's first line of defense against invaders includes the nose, mouth, eyes, lungs, and stomach. When the immune system reacts to an allergen, these body parts make great battlegrounds. Symptoms include runny nose; sneezing; watery, swollen, or red eyes; nasal congestion; wheezing; shortness of breath; a tight feeling in the chest; difficulty breathing; coughing; diarrhea; nausea; headache; fatigue; and a general feeling of misery. Symptoms can occur alone or in combination.

What Causes Allergies?

Blame your genes. The tendency to become allergic is inherited, and allergies typically develop before age 30. What you become allergic to is based on what substances you are exposed to and how often you are exposed to them. Generally, the more you are exposed to an allergen, the more likely it is to trigger a reaction. Unfortunately, there is no cure for allergies. But there are ways to ease your long-suffering sinuses and skin.

Traditional Remedies

Hot tea can act as a natural decongestant, with mint in particular producing good effects. Basil tea is another traditional remedy—not drunk, but used as a rinse on the skin.

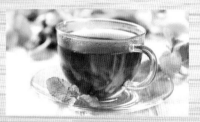

Turmeric

The curcumin in turmeric blocks the immune system from releasing histamine and acts as a decongestant, providing some relief from these symptoms.

In fact, research has shown that curcumin may reduce allergy symptoms by up to 70 percent, giving those who deal with seasonal allergies an effective, natural remedy without side effects. Adding a curcumin supplement to your daily routine during allergy season can work wonders, or try ending your day with some soothing turmeric milk to combat symptoms.

Taking Turmeric

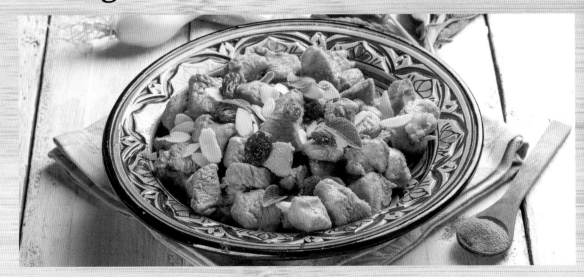

When we think of turmeric's earthy aroma and bright color, the first thing that comes to mind is probably curry and other Indian dishes. And ingesting the spice is certainly a popular way to reap its benefits, but there are several other methods for ingesting and using turmeric, as well. So let's look at a few ways that turmeric can spice up your daily life.

Eating and Drinking

Indian cuisine is one of those "love it or hate it" kinds of foods, with many people opting to avoid the spicy dishes. But if you fall into the "hate it" camp, don't discount turmeric altogether—the spice can be added to more than just curries! Sprinkle some on eggs, roasted vegetables, meats, or soups for extra flavor, or add a bit to a smoothie. You can also use the spice to make a flavorful broth, or try turmeric tea—also known as "golden milk"—for a comforting, warming beverage.

One thing to keep in mind when using turmeric in any recipe is the issue of bioavailability. Remember, curcumin has poor bioavailability unless it is paired with peperine, a substance found in black pepper. So always be sure to include a pinch of black pepper to increase curcumin's absorption. It's also smart to take turmeric along with a bit of fat, as curcumin is not very soluble in water but is fat soluble. Ayurvedic medicinal practices often suggest taking turmeric with ghee, a type of clarified butter. But there are many other healthy fats you can pair with the spice to ensure better bioavailability, such as coconut oil, olive oil, almonds, or avocado. Finally, studies have shown that heating turmeric can greatly increase the solubility of curcumin, and may even increase its antioxidant properties. So for maximum effectiveness when eating or drinking with the spice, add some pepper, include a fat, and apply heat!

Topical Turmeric

Turmeric's anti-inflammatory and antioxidant properties make it a perfect addition to skin-soothing
lotions and potions, which can help diminish acne,
soothe eczema, decrease muscle soreness, and
heal cuts and scrapes. You can find the ingredient in
many brand-name face creams and masks, and also
in pain-relieving salves and balms. But you can also
mix up your own curcumin concoctions with a few
simple ingredients.

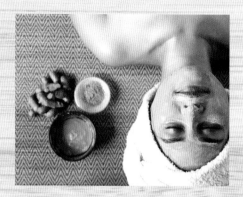

For instance, for an anti-inflammatory poultice, combine castor oil, turmeric, and a bit of
black pepper to make a thick paste, then apply to the inflamed area and keep it wrapped
with a bandage for several hours. Remember that turmeric easily stains, so when using the
spice topically, be sure to have some old towels on hand.

Supplements

Perhaps the easiest way to consume turmeric is through supplements. This is also a great choice if you simply don't like the taste of
the spice or if you'd rather avoid staining skin or clothes. And since
the curcumin content is premeasured and labeled, you don't need to
guess about whether you're ingesting the right amount of the spice.

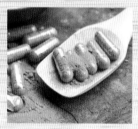

Experts recommend about 500 milligrams of curcumin a day to prevent chronic inflammation, which can easily be consumed in one or two supplement capsules. In contrast, there
are about 200 milligrams of curcumin in a teaspoon of ground turmeric, so you'd need to
eat at least two and a half teaspoons of the spice per day to get the same benefits. And
for joint inflammation and pain from disorders like arthritis, the recommended dosage is
between twice and four times that amount, so supplements are the clear winner in these
cases. As with other methods of ingestion, look for a supplement that includes black pepper or peperine, and take the supplements with a little bit of fat to aid absorption.

There is one exception to curcumin's bioavailability problem, and it concerns digestive disorders. If you take turmeric to aid irritable bowel syndrome or another digestive issue, you
don't have to worry about increasing the spice's bioavailability. When you ingest turmeric
for its digestive benefits, there's no need for it to be absorbed into the bloodstream, as the
spice automatically ends up in the area of the body where it is most beneficial: the digestive
system. Of course, with such a variety of uses and benefits, it might be worth a bit of effort
to get the most out of what turmeric can do.

Cautions

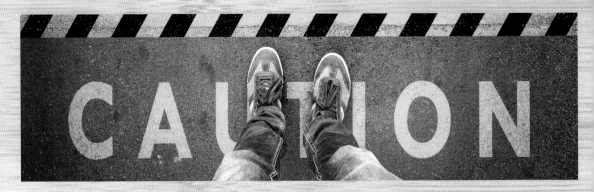

There's no doubt that turmeric exhibits a host of benefits, from its anti-inflammatory and antioxidant properties to its effects on the brain and blood vessels. What's more, the golden spice is opening up exciting possibilities for treatments of serious diseases and disorders. And it certainly doesn't hurt that turmeric is a delicious addition to many dishes, both savory and sweet, and provides a natural way to add a lovely hue to both foods and fabrics.

But all too often, when we hear the word "natural," we also assume unconditional safety; however, even natural ingredients must be used with a bit of caution. Turmeric is no exception. Although the spice is generally considered very safe and well-tolerated in most cases, there are some issues to be aware of.

Allergic Reactions

First, as with any other food, it should be noted that turmeric can cause allergic reactions. Since turmeric is a member of the ginger family, those who are allergic to plants in this family are the most susceptible. Also be cautious if you have an allergy to yellow food coloring, which is often derived from turmeric. Allergies can occur from ingestion as well as from topical application, and can include symptoms like hives, itching, and shortness of breath.

Large Dosages

Another issue to be mindful of is the dosage amount of turmeric. Although little research has been done on high doses of the spice, there is evidence that taking large amounts of it can result in an irregular heartbeat, upset stomach, dizziness, or diarrhea. Large doses of turmeric can also have the unfortunate effect of worsening certain symptoms. For instance, while its anti-inflammatory effects are known to lessen the pain of arthritis, too much turmeric can actually exacerbate arthritis symptoms. Large amounts of the spice can also worsen gallbladder, heartburn, and acid-reflux issues.

Kidney Stones

Turmeric contains a substance called oxalate, an organic compound found in many plants that can bind to minerals like iron and calcium in the digestive system or in the kidneys. When too much oxalate and calcium bind in the kidneys, they can form kidney stones. Although turmeric only contains about 2 percent oxalate, large amounts of the spice can lead to this painful condition, so for those who are prone to kidney stones, it's best to ingest turmeric sparingly.

Interactions

While the spice can help to lower high blood pressure and high blood sugar, those who already take medications for these conditions may want to avoid taking turmeric supplements, as the combination may lower blood pressure or blood sugar too much. In the same vein, turmeric may interfere with anti-inflammatory medications or cholesterol regulators, even though the spice has been shown to work as an anti-inflammatory and may help to lower cholesterol. So always check with your doctor before beginning a supplement regimen, especially if you take prescription medications.

Blood Thinning Effects

Another possible side effect from turmeric is an increased risk of bleeding, as the spice may slow blood clotting and act as a blood thinner. For this reason, it is important to avoid turmeric before any kind of surgery, and it should not be taken in supplement form during pregnancy. Blood thinning medication—including over-the-counter drugs that increase bleeding risk, like aspirin and ibuprofen—can react with turmeric and result in bruising or bleeding. The spice also increases the blood-thinning effect of certain herbal remedies, including angelica, clove, garlic, ginger, and gingko, so use caution if combining turmeric with other supplements.

Children

Finally, the safety of turmeric in children has not been studied or well documented. The possibility of bleeding, lowered blood pressure, and a weakened immune system exists for children who take the supplement, so it's smart to keep it away from younger family members altogether.

In short, while the benefits of turmeric are hard to deny, the spice is not without risk, as well. Be smart about dosage, double-check all medications, and most importantly, always discuss treatment and prevention plans with your doctor, even before using a "natural" remedy.

Traditional Golden Milk

- 2 cups milk
- 1 teaspoon grated fresh turmeric
- Freshly crushed black pepper, equal to 2-3 peppercorns
- Honey to taste

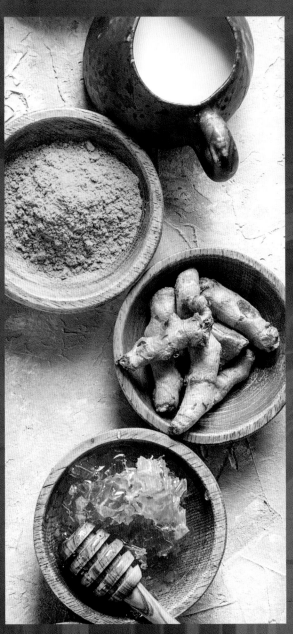

Golden milk is a turmeric-infused beverage that is associated with the ayurvedic tradition of India (as well as with other Asian countries). It is used to ward off illness and support the mind and body. Variations on the recipe have proliferated in recent years, but the basic ingredients consist of milk, turmeric, and honey. This preparation keeps it simple and traditional.

Heat all ingredients except honey in a saucepan and simmer covered for 10-15 minutes. Stir in honey and serve.

Makes 4 servings

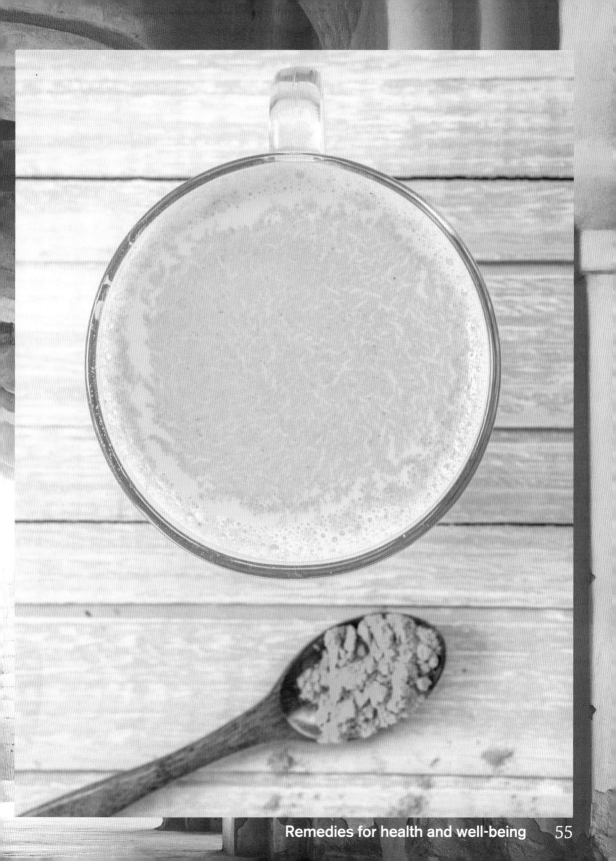

Thai Fried Rice

- 2½ cups water
- 1⅓ cups long-grain white rice
- 8 ounces ground pork or pork sausage (optional)
- 1 tablespoon vegetable oil
- 1 medium onion, thinly sliced
- 1 tablespoon finely chopped fresh ginger
- 1 jalapeño pepper,* seeded and finely chopped
- 3 cloves garlic, minced
- ½ teaspoon ground turmeric
- 2 tablespoons fish sauce
- 2 cups chopped cooked vegetables such as broccoli, zucchini, red bell peppers, carrots, bok choy or spinach
- 3 eggs, lightly beaten
- 3 green onions, thinly sliced
- ½ cup cilantro leaves

***Jalapeños can sting and irritate the skin, so wear rubber gloves when handling peppers and do not touch your eyes.

1. Bring water and rice to a boil in medium saucepan over high heat. Reduce heat to low; cover and simmer 20 minutes or until water is absorbed.

2. Fluff rice with fork. Let cool to room temperature. Cover and refrigerate until cold, at least 1 hour or up to 24 hours.

3. When rice is cold, cook pork in wok or medium skillet over medium-high heat until no longer pink. Drain off excess fat; transfer pork to bowl and set aside.

4. Heat wok or large skillet over medium-high heat. Add oil and swirl to coat surface. Add onion, ginger, jalapeño, garlic and turmeric; stir-fry 4 to 6 minutes or until onion is tender.

5. Stir in fish sauce; mix well. Stir in cold rice, vegetables and pork; cook and stir 3 to 4 minutes or until heated through.

6. Push rice mixture to side of wok and pour eggs into center. Cook eggs 2 to 3 minutes or just until set, lifting and stirring to scramble. Stir rice mixture into eggs.

7. Stir in green onions. Transfer to serving bowl; sprinkle with cilantro.

Makes 4 servings

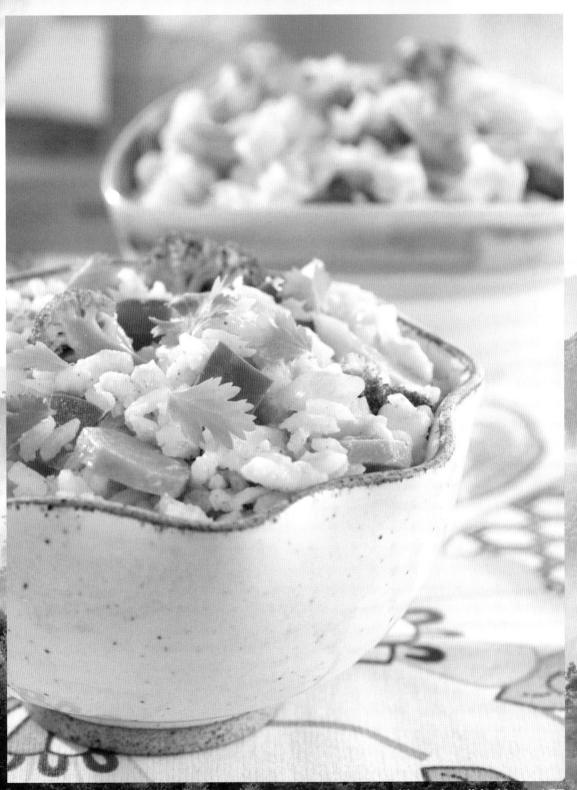

Moroccan Chickpeas

- 1 cup chopped onion
- ¼ cup reduced-sodium vegetable broth
- 2 cloves garlic, crushed
- 2 cans (about 15 ounces each) chickpeas, rinsed and drained
- 1 can (28 ounces) reduced-sodium diced tomatoes
- ½ cup sliced red bell pepper
- ½ cup sliced yellow bell pepper
- ½ cup sliced green bell pepper
- 2 tablespoons oil-cured olives, pitted and chopped
- 1 teaspoon ground cumin
- 1 teaspoon ground ginger
- 1 teaspoon ground turmeric
- 1 bay leaf
- 2 tablespoons lemon juice

1. Combine onion, broth and garlic in large nonstick skillet. Cook and stir over medium heat 3 minutes or until onion softens.

2. Add chickpeas, tomatoes, bell peppers, olives, cumin, ginger, turmeric and bay leaf. Stir well. Simmer 5 minutes or until bell peppers are tender. Remove and discard bay leaf. Stir in lemon juice; adjust seasonings.

Makes 6 servings

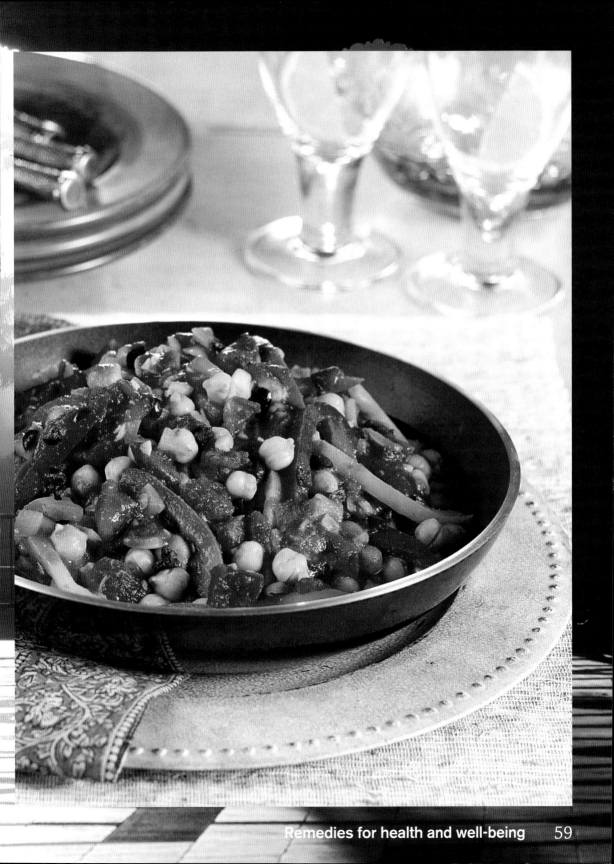

Mediterranean Fish Soup

- 4 ounces uncooked pastina or other small pasta
- ¾ cup chopped onion
- 2 cloves garlic, minced
- 1 teaspoon whole fennel seeds
- 1 can (about 14 ounces) no-salt-added stewed tomatoes
- 1 can (about 14 ounces) fat-free reduced-sodium chicken broth
- 1 tablespoon minced fresh Italian parsley
- ½ teaspoon black pepper
- ¼ teaspoon ground turmeric
- 8 ounces firm, white-fleshed fish, cut into 1-inch pieces
- 3 ounces small raw shrimp, peeled (with tails on)

1. Cook pasta according to package directions, omitting salt. Drain.

2. Spray large saucepan with nonstick cooking spray; heat over medium heat. Add onion, garlic and fennel seeds; cook and stir 3 minutes or until onion is crisp-tender.

3. Stir in tomatoes, broth, parsley, pepper and turmeric; bring to a boil. Reduce heat to low; simmer 10 minutes.

4. Stir fish into saucepan; cook 1 minute. Add shrimp; cook until shrimp are pink and opaque. Divide pasta evenly among 4 bowls; ladle soup evenly over pasta.

Makes 4 servings

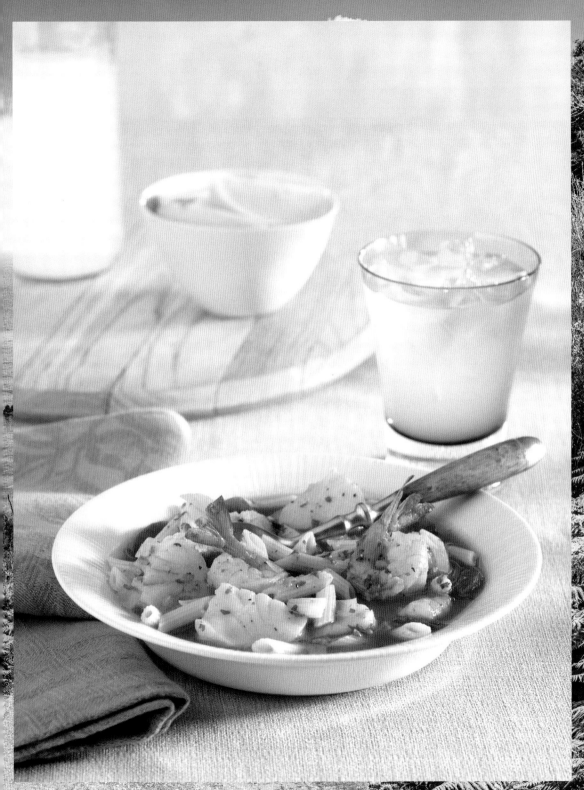

Shrimp and Chicken Paella

- ¾ cup cooked rice
- 2 cans (about 14 ounces each) no-salt-added diced tomatoes, divided
- ½ teaspoon ground turmeric
- 1 package (12 ounces) medium raw shrimp, peeled and deveined (with tails on)
- 2 chicken tenders (about 4 ounces), cut into 1-inch pieces
- 1 cup frozen peas

1. Preheat oven to 400°F. Lightly coat 8-inch square baking dish with nonstick cooking spray.

2. Spread rice in prepared baking dish. Pour 1 can of tomatoes over rice; sprinkle with turmeric. Arrange shrimp and chicken over tomatoes; top with peas.

3. Drain remaining can of tomatoes, discarding juice. Spread tomatoes evenly over shrimp and chicken.

4. Cover and bake 30 minutes. Let stand, covered, 5 minutes before serving.

Serving Suggestion: Serve with a green salad tossed with mustard vinaigrette and garnished with ½ cup corn kernels

Makes 4 servings

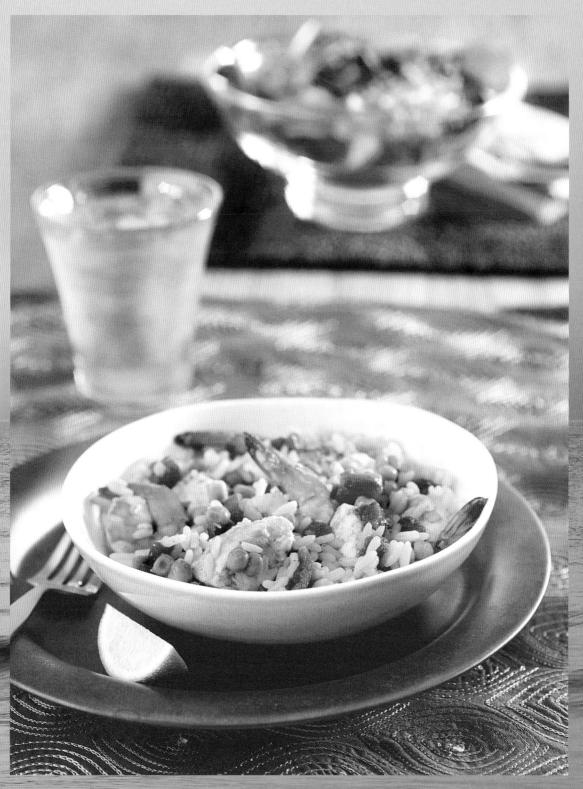

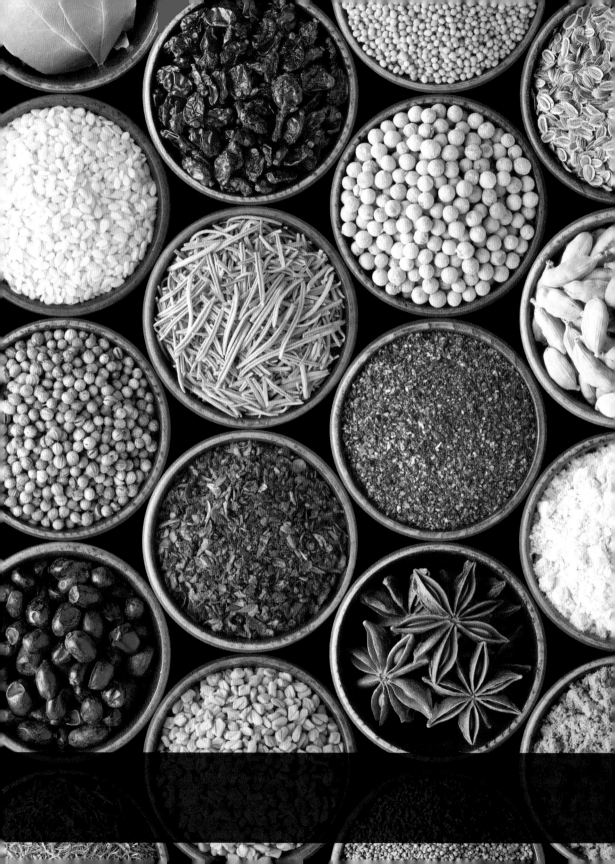

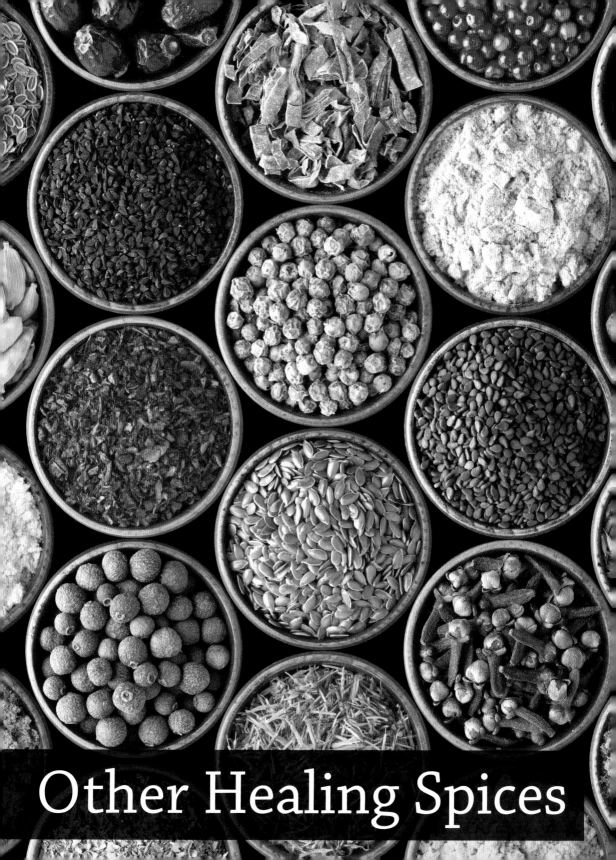

Other Healing Spices

Ajwain

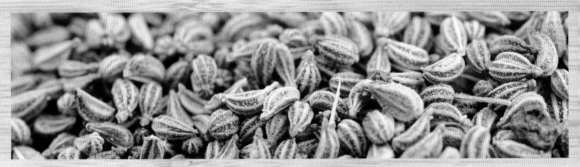

Ajwain—also known as ajowan, ajowan caraway, bishop's weed, and carom—is an annual herb from the Apiaceae (or Umbelliferae) family, to which caraway, cumin, and fennel also belong. Mostly cultivated in India, Pakistan, Afghanistan, Iran and Egypt, the herb's leaves and fruit are both edible and often used in Indian cooking. The greenish-brown, striped fruits of the plant are sometimes mistakenly called seeds, due to their small, dry appearance.

Ajwain fruits have a pungent aroma of thyme, as they contain an essential oil that is made up of 50 percent thymol—the same substance that is found in the evergreen herb. Dry roasting or frying the fruits in oil or ghee mellows the flavor of the spice somewhat, giving it a taste similar to oregano combined with anise. The fruits can also be ground or crushed, to release the oils and increase their flavor.

Use in Ayurvedic Medicine

In addition to its use in cuisine, the spice has traditionally been used in Ayurvedic medicine. The fruits are sold whole, and those who wish to use them medicinally will sometimes chew the small pods while raw, to address issues like indigestion, bloating, diarrhea, and fatigue. But chewing on the fruits in this way results in a bitter and hot flavor that can leave the tongue numb afterwards. Fortunately, it is not necessary to suffer unpleasant consequences to enjoy the benefits of this spice.

Health Benefits

And the benefits provided by ajwain are numerous: To begin with, the spice is a nutritional powerhouse, packing fiber, protein, minerals, and antioxidants into its tiny seed-like fruits. Ajwain has also been found to have antibacterial and antifungal properties. In addition to thymol, the spice's other main active compound is carvacrol. Thymol and carvacrol have both been proven to inhibit the growth of bacteria and fungi, including *E. coli* and *Salmonella*, two major food poisoning culprits. One study even found that ajwain was effective against antibiotic-resistant strains of bacteria, a finding which could greatly influence future medicine.

Ajwain is being studied for its effects on high cholesterol and high blood pressure, as well, although further research is needed to confirm this. But preliminary research in animals has shown that high concentrations of the fruit's extract significantly lowers cholesterol and triglycerides. Similarly, studies in rats have shown that ajwain lowers blood pressure levels. While the effects on humans have yet to be researched, the possibilities look hopeful!

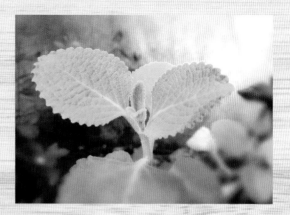

Traditional Remedies

Traditionally, ajwain has been used as a household remedy for indigestion, ulcers, and asthma, and the pods are crushed and applied as a poultice to relieve arthritis. While these effects haven't been formally studied in humans, centuries of anecdotal evidence have made the spice a popular medicinal ingredient in India and Sri Lanka.

Ideas for Use

To avoid the tongue-numbing effects of the spice, it is best to pan roast or fry it first, so the taste will be milder. Ajwain works well in savory dishes with vegetables or lentils, and is often used in starchy foods like bread. It can also be used as a pickling spice, as a way to season chicken or fish, or it can be ground up and mixed with other spices to create a curry powder.

But a surprising way to ingest this spice is by making "ajwain water," a popular medicinal remedy in India. To make it, just add two teaspoons of dry roasted ajwain to a cup of water and allow it to sit overnight (or, if you're in a hurry, boil the mixture, strain, and wait for it to cool). In the morning, simply mix the water and strain it. It's then ready to drink. Experts recommend drinking the water on an empty stomach, and say it helps with digestion and prevents acid reflux. Some even claim that the beverage promotes weight loss, thanks to its ability to regulate digestion.

Cautions

Ajwain is offering some exciting possibilities to the world of natural remedies. Just be sure not to overdo it—consuming large amounts of the spice has been known to cause nausea. And of course, women who are pregnant or breastfeeding should consult their doctor before consuming the spice, to be sure it's safe. While many of ajwain's purported benefits still need to be studied, there is no doubt that adding these tiny pods to your spice rack is a smart move.

Allspice

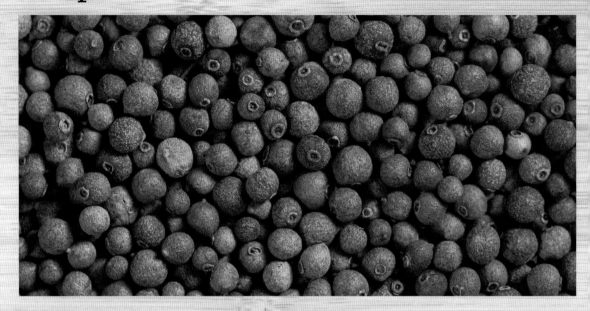

You might think allspice is a mix of spices, but it comes from the dried fruit of a single ever-green plant, *Pimenta dioica*. Unripe rather than mature fruit is used to create the spice. The name was coined sometime in the early 17th century, thanks to the spice's rich notes of cinnamon, clove, cardamom, nutmeg, and pepper.

Where Is It Grown?

Used in Caribbean cooking under the name pimento, allspice originated in the Caribbean region, southern Mexico, and Central America. Its popularity has spread, and it's also a popular spice in Middle Eastern cuisine and in seasonal deserts in the U.S. And residents of Cincinnati, Ohio, will recognize the flavor of allspice from their iconic chili.

Health Benefits

The plant's benefits go beyond food: the essential oil is prized for many health and beauty uses. Allspice oil contains antioxidant compounds including methyl eugenol and cineol, as well as vitamins A, B, and C. This makes it excellent for fighting oxidative stress in the body. Allspice is used in folk medicine for its reputed ability to ease diarrhea, indigestion, and vomiting, as well as menstrual cramps and the symptoms of menopause. A 2009 study into the use of herbal medicines taken by Costa Rican menopausal women noted that plant extracts from *Pimenta dioica* did bind with estrogen receptors, suggesting a mechanism through which the spice might work to treat menopause symptoms, though it also called for more research on its potential.

Ideas for Use

Like cloves, which also contain eugenol, allspice has a reputation for relieving toothache. Wet your finger and dip it into the spice—not the essential oil—then rub it along the gum line near the aching tooth. You can also steep some in a glass of warm water, then rinse your mouth with it. Not only does this rinse relieve pain, it also freshens your breath. (In fact, allspice is used commercially to flavor toothpaste.)

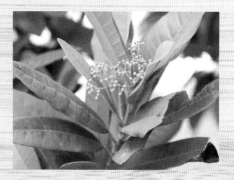

The oil can be used to treat wounds and prevent infections. When rubbed into joints and muscles, its analgesic effects provide soothing relief for arthritis, muscle strains, and insect bites. Allspice should always be used with a carrier oil, as it can be irritating to the skin when undiluted.

A few drops of the essential oil mixed with sugar and coconut oil create an aromatic face scrub.

MOROCCAN SPICED HONEY SOAP TRAVEL-SIZE REFRESHING BODY WASH

- 1 pound honey soap base
- 6 drops allspice oil
- 6 drops cardamom oil
- 6 drops cinnamon oil
- 6 drops clove essential oil
- Dried bay leaves
- Soap molds
- Coconut oil

Grease soap molds with coconut oil. Cut soap base into chunks, and melt in a double boiler or in the microwave (heating for 20-second intervals and stirring the soap in between intervals). Remove from heat and mix in all essential oils. Place a bay leaf in each mold, and fill with mixture. Allow to set for two hours before removing from molds.

With its bay leaf accent, this soap is pretty enough to place in a guest bathroom. Allspice, cardamom, cinnamon, and clove essential oils team up to provide a spicy scent and plenty of antiseptic and antioxidant benefits. Look for a melt and pour soap base with honey, which is a natural humectant and helps skin retain moisture.

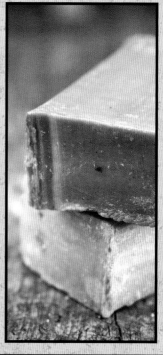

White Bean Chili

- ¾ cup cooked rice
- 1 pound ground chicken
- 3 cups coarsely chopped celery
- 1½ cups coarsely chopped onions (about 2 medium)
- 3 cloves garlic, minced
- 4 teaspoons chili powder
- 1½ teaspoons ground cumin
- ¾ teaspoon ground allspice
- ¾ teaspoon ground cinnamon
- ½ teaspoon black pepper
- 1 can (16 ounces) whole tomatoes, undrained and coarsely chopped
- 1 can (about 15 ounces) Great Northern beans, rinsed and drained
- 2 cups fat-free reduced-sodium chicken broth

1. Spray large nonstick skillet with nonstick cooking spray; heat over medium heat. Add chicken; cook and stir until browned, breaking into pieces. Remove chicken; drain fat from skillet.

2. Add celery, onions and garlic to skillet; cook and stir over medium heat 5 to 7 minutes or until tender. Sprinkle with chili powder, cumin, allspice, cinnamon and pepper; cook and stir 1 minute.

3. Return chicken to skillet. Stir in tomatoes with juice, beans and broth; bring to a boil. Reduce heat to low. Simmer, uncovered, 15 minutes.

Makes 6 servings

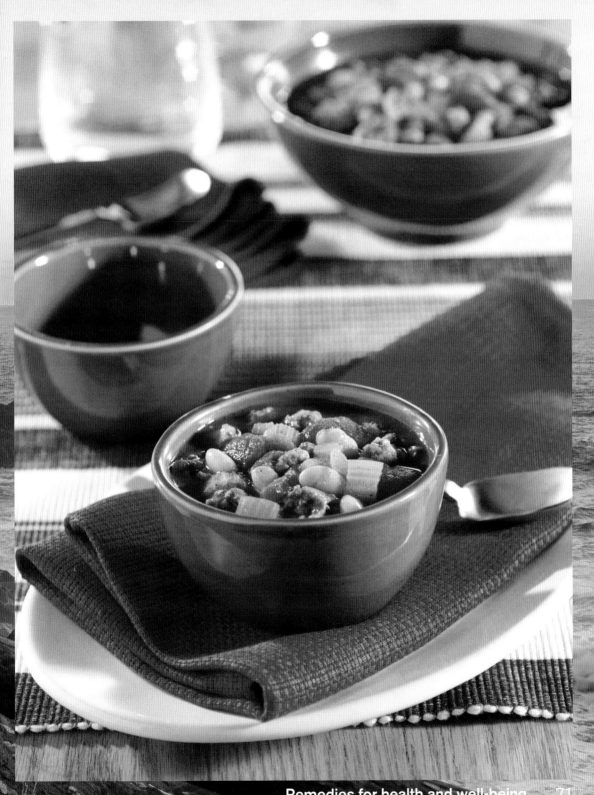

Asafetida

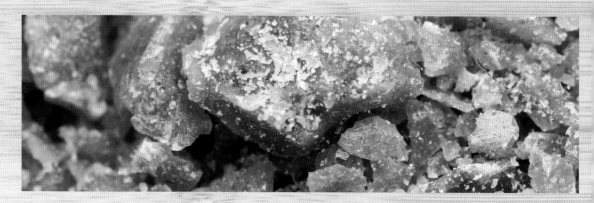

With a nickname like "devil's dung," it's a wonder anyone ever gave asafetida an honored place in the world of spices. But this dried resin, which is extracted from the root of a perennial herb, has been used medicinally as far back as 700 B.C. The spice is also used in cooking, which may seem surprising considering its pungent smell, which has been likened to spoiled garlic, cooked cabbage, and even manure. In fact, asafetida (also spelled "asafoetida") can be literally translated from Latin as "stinking gum."

History

A member of the carrot family, asafetida is native to Iran and Afghanistan, but today is mostly grown in India. It is believed to be similar to an extinct plant known as silphium, which was used as a medicine and spice in antiquity. When silphium began to die off due to overzealous harvesting practices, a plant was sought which could replicate its medicinal properties. Asafetida, despite its unpleasant aroma, was thought to be a suitable replacement, even receiving the blessing of Alexander the Great, who introduced the spice to Europe.

While this "stinking gum" may exude an unappetizing smell when raw—the odor is so strong that it can permeate other nearby spices if not stored in an airtight container—asafetida undergoes a dramatic transformation when it is cooked. Sautéing the spice in oil or ghee softens the pungent aroma and results in a flavor similar to shallots or leeks, which provides dishes with a savory umami component.

The spice has also been used in a variety of other ways, such as a wildlife repellant and moth trap bait, and has been an element of folk magic in several cultures, where it has been used to prevent illness, repel evil spirits, and protect from demonic forces. It was even used in the Old West as a cure for alcoholism. But asafetida's transforming flavor, repellent nature, and curative properties are secondary to the long list of health benefits the spice provides.

Health Benefits

Traditionally, asafetida was used to treat respiratory issues due to asthma, bronchitis, and the flu; digestive disorders like indigestion, nausea, and gas; illnesses like whooping cough and croup; and nervous conditions like hysteria and insanity. Nowadays, the spice is still prized for its antispasmodic and carminative properties that help to improve digestion and lessen symptoms of irritable bowel syndrome, and it is also thought to protect against high cholesterol and triglycerides. Asafetida may have anti-inflammatory, antibacterial, and expectorant properties, so it is still recommended for lung-related issues like asthma.

The spice contains a substance called coumarin, which is a natural blood thinner, and researchers have discovered that it can significantly reduce blood pressure as well as prevent blood clots. What's more, studies in animals have shown that asafetida can help maintain blood sugar levels. This finding could potentially lead to new treatments for diabetes.

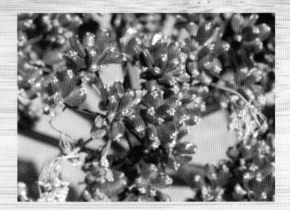

Ideas for Use

The spice is not often found in neighborhood grocery stores, but those who wish to try it can easily purchase it online or at Middle Eastern or Indian grocery stores. It is often sold as a powder, but can also be found in larger chunks which must be ground or grated before use. Don't be put off by its strong, pungent smell—cooking the spice will mellow the flavor and give dishes a savory onion-like flavor.

Although asafetida has been used medicinally for millennia, most of the evidence of its benefits is still anecdotal. As a result, there is no clinical evidence to support recommended dosages. Still, the spice is available in supplement form for those who want to test out its reported benefits, with a daily dosage between 200 and 500 milligrams being traditionally prescribed.

Cautions

As it is known to be a blood thinner, asafetida should be avoided by anyone with a bleeding disorder or who takes anticoagulants, and it should not be taken for at least two weeks prior to surgery. It has also been known to interact with high blood pressure medication, and should never be taken by women who are pregnant or breastfeeding or by children, except in the small amounts that would normally be found in food.

Black Pepper

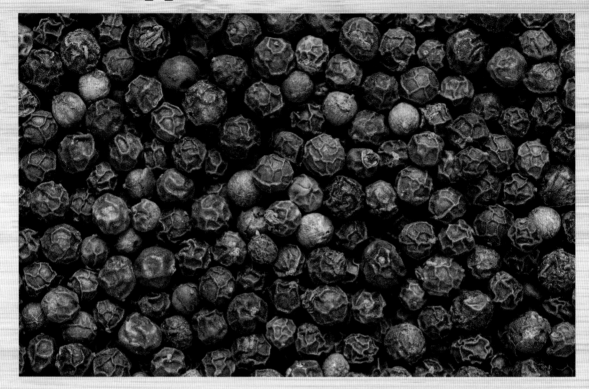

Traded more than any other spice in the world, black pepper has been prized since antiquity not only for its flavor-enhancing spiciness, but also for its medicinal usefulness. The spice has been found in ancient Egyptian tombs, was frequently used in ancient Roman cookery, and was so coveted by Europeans that it was briefly used as a form of currency. In fact, Alaric the Visigoth, famous for sacking the city of Rome in the year 410, demanded 3,000 pounds of pepper as a ransom for the city! The spice is obtained by cooking and drying the unripe fruit of the flowering vine. Once dried, oil can be extracted from the fruit by crushing it.

Health Benefits

Some studies have shown that using black pepper in marinades used on beef can help reduce the carcinogens that can develop in beef when it is cooked at high temperatures. An active ingredient in black pepper, piperine can help the body absorb other helpful chemicals—including the curcumin found in turmeric, as well as a compound called resveratrol found in red wine. Some have also claimed that black pepper can help aid digestion. There have not been sufficient large-scale studies done on humans to determine whether all the health benefits apply when the spice is used in the quantities used in cooking.

Folk Remedies

If you're suffering from PMS, add a pinch to 1 tablespoon aloe vera gel, and take three times a day with meals to relieve symptoms such as backache and abdominal pain.

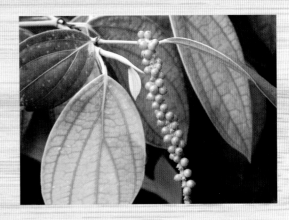

Pepper is a bit of an irritant (try sniffling some), but this characteristic is a plus for those suffering from coughs accompanied by thick mucus. The irritating property of pepper stimulates circulation and the flow of mucus in the airways and sinuses. Place 1 teaspoon black pepper into a cup and sweeten things up with the addition of 1 tablespoon honey. Fill with boiling water, steep for 10 to 15 minutes, stir, and sip.

Black Pepper Essential Oil

In the form of essential oil, black pepper is said to supports cell function, immune system, and circulation; act as an antioxidant; and provide a warming sensation when applied topically.

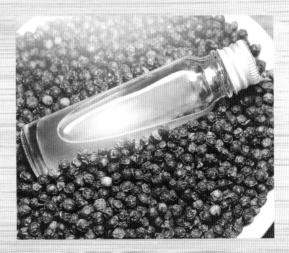

The warming properties of black pepper oil make it ideal for soothing sore muscles and aiding in relief from arthritis and rheumatism. A couple diluted drops rubbed into the affected area can help improve pain and ease mobility. Taken internally (again, diluted), black pepper oil protects the body from free radicals and helps to repair cell damage, and has even been shown to lower cholesterol. It may also aid digestion, and help to kill harmful bacteria in the body.

Cautions

Black pepper oil should not be taken in large quantities, as it can cause vomiting, sleeplessness, and overheating. Also, care should be used when applying topically, as the warming sensation of the oil may be irritating for sensitive skin.

Shepherd's Pie Potatoes

- 4 large russet potatoes (about 12 ounces each)
- 1½ tablespoons olive oil, divided
- 3 to 4 tablespoons milk
- 2 tablespoons butter
- 1 teaspoon salt, divided
- ½ teaspoon black pepper, divided
- 1 small onion, chopped
- 1 carrot, chopped
- 1 clove garlic, minced
- 12 ounces ground beef chuck
- 2 tablespoons tomato paste
- 1 tablespoon Worcestershire sauce
- 1/2 teaspoon ground thyme
- ½ cup water
- ½ cup thawed frozen peas

1. Preheat oven to 400°F. Scrub potatoes; prick all over with fork. Brush with 1 tablespoon oil; place on baking sheet. Bake about 1 hour or until fork-tender.

2. Cut ¼-inch slice from top of each potato. Scoop out flesh into medium bowl, leaving ¼-inch shells. Add 3 tablespoons milk, butter, ½ teaspoon salt and ¼ teaspoon pepper; mash until smooth, adding additional milk if necessary. Return potato shells to baking sheet.

3. While potatoes are baking, heat remaining ½ tablespoon oil in large skillet over medium-high heat. Add onion and carrot; cook about 8 minutes or until vegetables are soft and beginning to brown, stirring occasionally. Add garlic; cook and stir 1 minute. Add beef; cook about 5 minutes or until no longer pink, stirring to break up meat. Add tomato paste, Worcestershire sauce, thyme and remaining ½ teaspoon salt and ¼ teaspoon pepper; cook and stir 2 minutes. Stir in water. Reduce heat to medium-low; cook about 10 minutes or until mixture thickens slightly, stirring occasionally. Stir in peas; cook 1 minute.

4. Divide beef mixture evenly among potato shells. Pipe or spread mashed potato mixture over beef mixture. (There may be extra mashed potatoes; serve on the side or reserve for another use.)

5. Bake about 20 minutes or until top of potatoes begin to brown.

Makes 4 servings

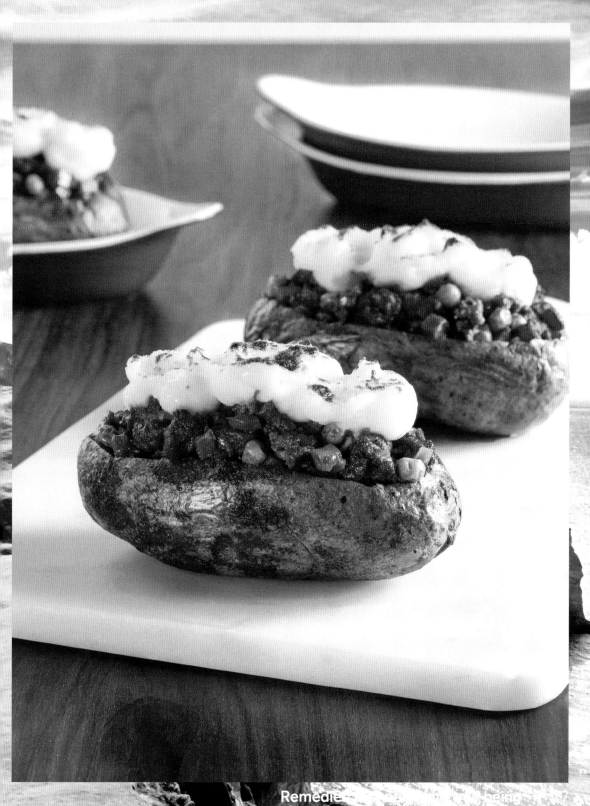

Caraway

Caraway, a biennial plant native to Asia, Europe, and North Africa, is no doubt best known for its culinary use. With its licorice-like flavor and aroma, the spice is commonly used in breads, desserts, and liquors throughout many world cultures.

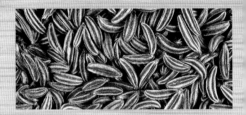

Related to parsley, caraway has become naturalized in North America. Caraway grows best in a light, average, well-drained soil in full sun, although it tolerates partial shade. Plant in place; caraway produces a long taproot and does not transplant easily.

A Long History

Fossilized caraway seeds have been found at Neolithic and Mesolithic archeological sites, proving that the spice has been in use for at least 8,000 years! Its use in folk medicine, especially as a digestive aid, has been documented since the time of ancient Egypt and Rome. This versatile spice was thought to cure colic in the young and gout in the old. The spice also had some, well, guard-dog qualities. Caraway was believed to protect objects from theft.

Historically, caraway has been used as a moth repellent.

Caraway Essential Oil

Caraway's strong aroma comes from its essential oil, which is distilled from the seeds and used to fragrance soaps, lotions, and perfumes. The essential oil is also added to mouthwashes and used to flavor liqueurs in Germany, Scandinavia, and Russia.

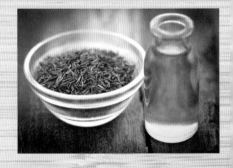

Ideas for Use

As a medicine, caraway is used—most often as a cordial—to relieve an upset stomach and dispel gas. But you may be most familiar with caraway from eating sauerkraut, rye crackers, and rye bread—foods that rely heavily on its strong aroma and taste. Add caraway seeds to beef dishes, stews, and breads. Add leaves to salads and soups. The herb complements eggs, cheese, sauces, barley, oats, pork, and fish, as well as cabbage, beets, spinach, potatoes, peas, cauliflower, turnips, and zucchini. Cooking it a long time can make it bitter, so add caraway no more than 30 minutes before a dish is done. It also makes children's medicines more tasty.

Folk Remedies

The most popular way to use caraway medicinally is in food. It is rare to find anyone using it by itself as a tincture or tea, but sometimes it flavors tinctures or syrups. Caraway can help prevent both internal and external infections, and can be used as a natural antihistamine. Its usefulness as a digestive aid has been known for millennia, as it helps to ease indigestion and heartburn, speeds up digestion, and protects the stomach from ulcers.

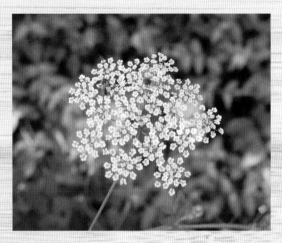

Caraway water has long been given to babies with colic.

A compress soaked in a strong infusion or the powdered and moistened seed relieves swelling and bruising.

For belching, try some caraway seeds, straight or sprinkled on a salad. They calm the digestive tract.

For flatulence, caraway seeds and their oils are carminatives (they get rid of gas), but who wants to eat just the seeds? Caraway seed crackers and breads with caraway seeds are a tasty way to make your system gas-unfriendly.

For occasional stomach upset, you can either make a tea from the seed or you can do what people in Middle Eastern countries have done for centuries—simply chew on the seeds after dinner.

Caraway seed tea

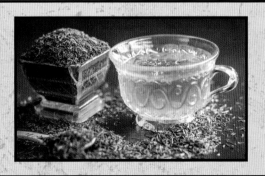

- Place 1 teaspoon caraway seeds in a cup and add boiling water.
- Cover the cup and let stand for ten minutes.
- Strain well and drink up to 3 cups a day—be sure to drink on an empty stomach

Reuben Rolls

- 1 cup sauerkraut
- 1 package (about 14 ounces) refrigerated pizza dough
- 6 thin slices Swiss cheese (about 4 ounces)
- 1 teaspoon caraway seeds
- ½ teaspoon black pepper
- 1/3 pound thinly sliced corned beef
- ½ cup Thousand Island dressing

1. Preheat oven to 400°F. Line baking sheet with parchment paper. Squeeze sauerkraut as dry as possible to yield about 2/3 cup.

2. Unroll dough on clean work surface or cutting board; press into 13X9-inch rectangle. Arrange cheese slices over dough, leaving 1 inch border on all sides. Sprinkle with sauerkraut, caraway seeds and pepper. Top with corned beef.

3. Starting with long side, gently roll up dough jelly-roll style. Trim off ends. Cut crosswise into eight 1½-inch slices with serrated knife; place slices cut sides up on prepared baking sheet.

4. Bake 20 to 25 minutes or until dough is golden brown and cheese is melted. Immediately remove from baking sheet; serve warm with dressing for dipping.

Makes 8 servings

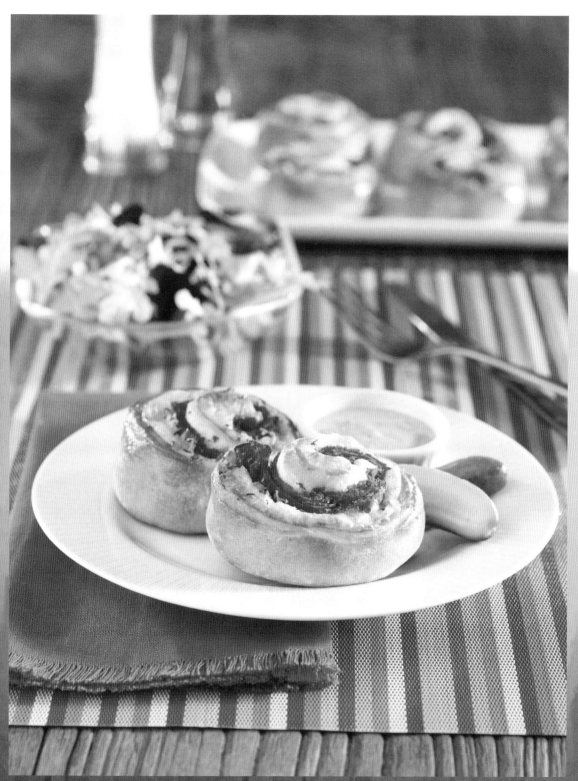

Cardamom

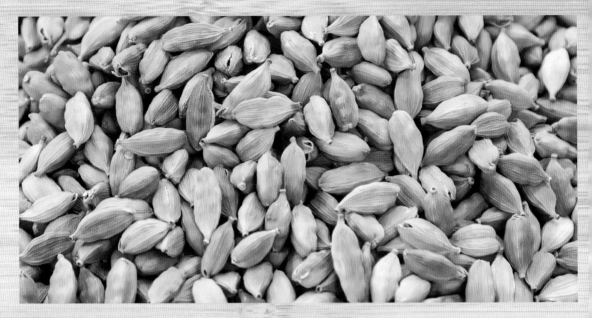

If you've ever sipped a cup of spicy chai tea or enjoyed Arabic coffee, they were probably flavored with a healthy dose of cardamom. The third most expensive spice in the world—only vanilla and saffron surpass it—cardamom is native to India; but it is surprisingly widespread in Nordic countries, as well, where it is used in traditional sweet buns and cakes. The spice may have found its way to Scandinavia when Vikings encountered it in Constantinople. And today, Swedes use 60 percent more cardamom than Americans.

Ideas for Use

Chewing on the seeds of aromatic spices such as clove, cardamom, or fennel after meals is a common practice in South Asia and the Middle East. The seeds of these spices contain antimicrobial properties that can help halt bad breath.

Cardamom seeds speed digestion. Add them to sautéed vegetables or to rice or lentils before cooking. You can also chew whole pods or steep pods in boiling water for several minutes to make a tea.

To relieve acid indigestion, add cardamom to baked goodies such as sweet rolls or fruit cake, or sprinkle, with a pinch of cinnamon, on toast. It works well in cooked cereals, too. You can also drink 1 cup papaya juice (it contains a natural, indigestion-fighting enzyme called papain) combined with 1 teaspoon sugar and 2 pinches cardamom. Warning! Pregnant women should not eat papayas; they're a source of natural estrogen that can cause miscarriage.

Folk Remedies

Add cardamom to massage oil and rub over the abdomen to relieve gas. Warmed olive and sesame oils are wonderful for massages.

To relieve nausea, chew 1 to 2 cardamom seeds. Another cardamom cure is to mix 2 pinches ground cardamom and ½ teaspoon honey into ½ cup plain yogurt. It will relieve nausea, and it's also a nutritious food to eat when you can't keep anything else down.

Cardamom seeds are also said to bust stress. To make a tea, cover 2 to 3 pods with boiling water and steep for ten minutes. Cardamom pods can be added to a regular pot of tea, too, in order to derive the calming effect. Also, crush the pods and add to rice or lentils before cooking, or use in a vegetable stirfry.

Instead of pods, you can use 1 teaspoon powdered cardamom, which is available in the spice section of the grocery store.

Essential Oil

Cardamom has soothing properties that make it great for aiding digestion and calming stomach upset. Try inhaling the scent on car or boat trips to ward off motion sickness. Used in aromatherapy, cardamom is said to help to relieve anxiety and promote feelings of calm. If a recipe calls for cardamom, the essential oil can be used in place of ground cardamom—a drop or two should be all you need!

Pick me up combo
- 8 drops lemon oil
- 2 drops eucalyptus oil
- 2 drops peppermint oil
- 1 drop cinnamon leaf oil
- 1 drop cardamom oil
- 2 ounces carrier oil

Combine the ingredients. Use as a massage oil, add 2 teaspoons to your bath, or add 1 teaspoon to a footbath. Without the carrier oil, this combination can be used in an aromatherapy diffuser, simmering pan of water, or a potpourri cooker, or it can be added to 2 ounces of water for an air spray. Use it as often as you like.

Nausea inhalation remedy
- 20 drops bergamot oil
- 20 drops cardamom oil
- 20 drops grapefruit oil
- 15 drops spearmint oil
- 10 drops geranium oil
- 3 drops ginger oil

Combine all ingredients in a small glass bottle. When you're feeling nauseous, shake the bottle and take a few whiffs.

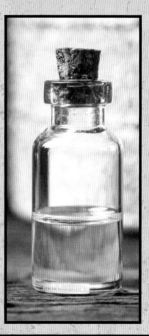

Chai Tea

- 2 quarts (8 cups) water
- 8 bags black tea
- ¾ cup sugar
- 16 whole cloves
- 16 whole cardamom seeds, pods removed
- 5 cinnamon sticks
- 8 slices fresh ginger
- 1 cup milk

1. Combine water, tea bags, sugar, cloves, cardamom, cinnamon sticks and ginger in slow cooker. Cover; cook on HIGH 2 to 2½ hours.

2. Strain mixture; discard solids. (At this point, tea may be covered and refrigerated up to 3 days.)

3. Stir in milk just before serving. Serve warm or chilled.

Makes 8 to 10 servings

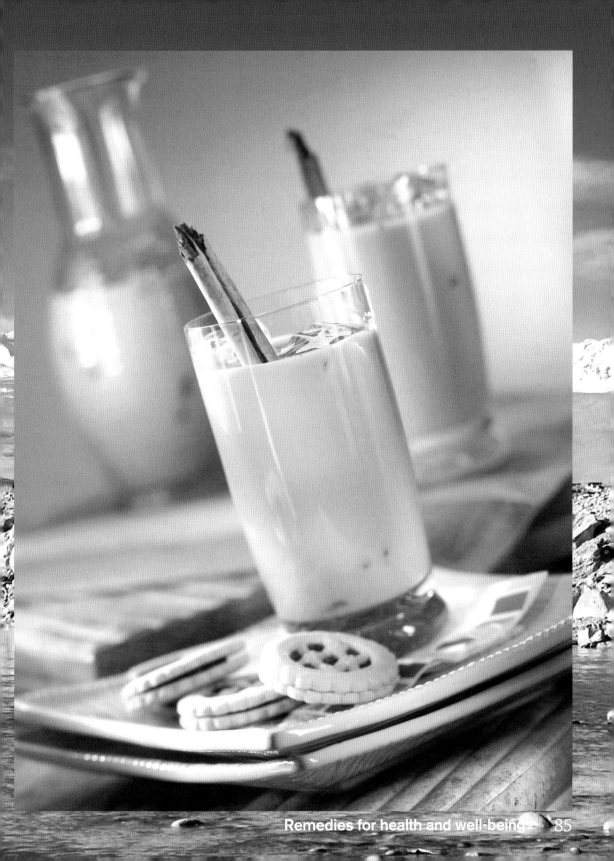

Cayenne Pepper

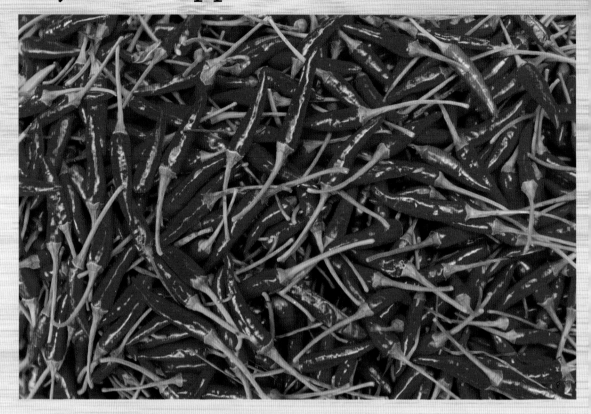

The fruits of these chili peppers are ground to make the powder. Cayenne peppers rate from 30,000 to 50,000 on the Scoville scale that measures the "heat" of spicy foods, spicier than the Jalapeno pepper but not nearly as hot as the habanero.

Cayenne grows naturally in the tropics, but gardeners in most parts of the United States can grow it with success. Cayenne's angular branches and stems may look purplish. Its red fruits are extremely hot. Flowers, which appear in drooping clusters on long stems, are star-shaped and yellowish-white. Leaves are long and elliptical.

You can grow it yourself! Unless you live in an area that rarely experiences freezing temperatures, it's best to plant cayenne in containers you can bring inside when temperatures drop, or grow it as an annual. The plant grows best in rich soil. If your soil is average, fertilize it with compost, rock phosphate, or wood ashes. Cayenne likes full sun. Give your plants lots of water during early stages of growth. Mulching protects them from drought. Pick cayenne peppers after the fruits have turned red. Dry immediately and store in a cool, dry place. You can also freeze cayenne peppers or preserve them in oil or vinegar.

Capsaicin

The main ingredient in cayenne is capsaicin, a powerful stimulant responsible for the pepper's heat. Although it can set your mouth on fire, cayenne, ironically, is good for your digestive system and is now known to help heal ulcers. It reduces substance P, a chemical that carries pain messages from the skin's nerve endings, so it reduces pain when applied topically. A cayenne cream is now in use to treat psoriasis, postsurgical pain, shingles, and nerve damage from diabetes. It may even help you burn off extra pounds. Researchers in England have found that about ¼ ounce of cayenne burns from 45 to 76 calories by increasing metabolism. Taking cayenne internally stabilizes blood pressure. You can apply powdered, dry cayenne as a poultice over wounds to stop bleeding. And in the kitchen, cayenne spices up any food it touches. Cayenne is also the source for the infamous "pepper spray," used by both the public and many police forces.

Health Benefits

Capsaicin creams are often recommended for those suffering from osteoarthritis, rheumatoid arthritis, and fibromyalgia. Numerous studies have shown that it can provide pain relief with relatively few side effects (some patients experienced burning at the application site.) Capsaicin ointment, 0.025 percent, is available over the counter.

For those suffering from psoriasis, studies have found that a cream containing capsaicin helped relieve itching and got rid of psoriasis plaques. Look for a cream containing 0.025 to 0.075 percent capsaicin—any more than that and you risk burning your skin. It takes about a week for the cream to work.

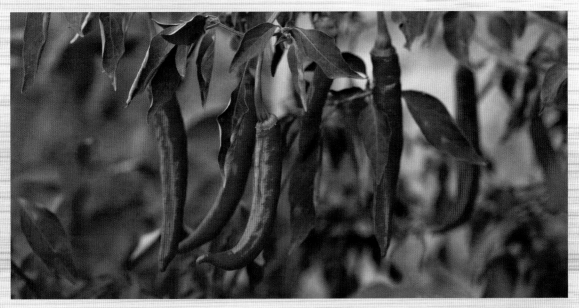

Ideas for Use

A dry mouth often inhibits taste buds from distinguishing between sour, sweet, salty, and bitter flavors. A mouthwatering method to stimulate saliva production and bolster those buds is to sprinkle red pepper (cayenne) on your food or mix it into your favorite juice (tomato juice seems most compatible). Better yet, prepare an entire meal around red pepper, which acts as nature's wake-up call, stimulating salivary glands, sweat glands, and tear ducts. Go south of the border with some spicy salsas or make that all-American favorite, chili, and start drooling!

When you're suffering from poor appetite, nothing revs up the old digestive engine like cayenne. Cayenne pepper has the power to make any dish fiery hot, but it also has a subtle flavor-enhancing quality. There is some evidence that eating hot pepper increases metabolism and the appetite. Add a few shakes of cayenne pepper to potato salad, deviled eggs, chili, and other hot dishes such as stews and soups.

Folk Remedies

Add a pinch of cayenne powder to other herbal infusions to treat colds and influenza. Simmer 3 tablespoons cayenne in 1 cup of cider vinegar. Do not strain. Shake before using. Take 1 teaspoon (4 droppers full) straight or add it to ½ cup warm water or tea for colds, flu, or sore throat. You can also combine cayenne with other heating herbs such as peppermint, eucalyptus, cinnamon, rosemary, and thyme in liniments for sore muscles or lung congestion.

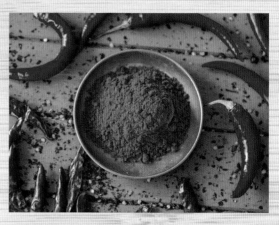

Cayenne pepper pulls no punches in delivering a hot and healing back pain remedy. To make a cayenne back rub to help with back pain, place 1 ounce cayenne pepper into 1 pint boiling water. Simmer for 30 minutes, remove from heat, and add a pint of rubbing alcohol. Cool and use when needed.

You can also make a pepper poultice by mixing cayenne pepper with flour and water to form a paste. Spread onto muslin, wrap up, and apply to the back.

Warning! Never apply cayenne pepper directly to the skin or you may suffer a burn or blisters. Do not touch your eyes while handling cayenne pepper, and always wash your hands well after handling peppers of any sort. Better yet, wear disposable rubber gloves.

CAPSAICIN CANDY

For a candy that will relieve canker sore pain, melt 1 pound caramels. Add ½ teaspoon cayenne pepper. Mix well and drop by teaspoonful onto waxed paper. Use this recipe for relief of mouth sores from chemotherapy and radiation, too. Be careful, though, as this may be too irritating for some people.

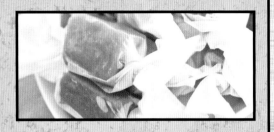

The fiery spice is a popular home treatment for mild high blood pressure. Cayenne pepper allows smooth blood flow by preventing platelets from clumping together and accumulating in the blood. Add some cayenne pepper to salt-free seasonings, or add a dash to a salad or in salt-free soups.

Used moderately, a little cayenne pepper can go a long way in helping ulcers. The pepper stimulates blood flow to bring nutrients to the stomach. To make a cup of peppered tea, mix ¼ teaspoon cayenne pepper in 1 cup hot water. Drink a cup a day. A dash of cayenne pepper can also be added to soups, meats, and other savory dishes.

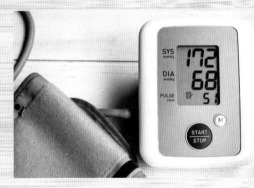

To warm cold feet, sprinkle a little cayenne pepper in your socks. However, this can be irritating to the skin after awhile, so carry some spare socks in case you need to change.

Cluster headaches can be quite severe and require special treatment. Try a cream made from capsaicin. Spread it on your forehead, temples, or any other area where you experience pain, but not too close to the eyes. The cream works best as a preventative, keeping the headache from forming in the first place. It needs to be applied four to five times a day for about four weeks to do much good, yet it is well worth the trouble.

Cautions

Overexposure to the skin can produce pain, dizziness, and a rapid pulse. Alcohol or fat, such as whole milk, neutralizes the reaction. If you touch a pepper and then rub your eyes or nose, you could inflame those sensitive tissues.

Chia Seed

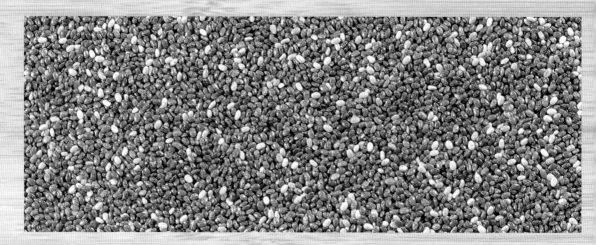

Is there anyone who hasn't seen a commercial for a Chia Pet (or possibly owned one)? These terra cotta figurines in the shape of bears, puppies, frogs—and even presidents!—are covered with tiny seeds, and within a few weeks they grow green "fur" or "hair" made of chia sprouts. A fun (if not slightly bizarre) novelty, to be certain; but those little chia seeds deserve to step out of the novelty shadows and have their moment in the superfood spotlight.

What Are Chia Seeds?

Chia seeds are edible seeds that come from the *Saliva hispanica* plant, a flowering, annual herb in the mint family. The plant is native to southern Mexico and Guatemala, where the word "chia" was derived from the Aztec word *chian* meaning "oily." It's a fitting name, as the seeds are rich in omega-3 fatty acids. Chia seeds are also uniquely hydrophilic, meaning they are attracted to water, and they can hold up to 12 times their weight in liquid. When the seeds are soaked, they develop a gelatinous coating and a distinctive texture, and this gelatin-like substance can be used in vegan recipes as an egg substitute.

Packed with Nutrition

In addition to its native countries, chia is now also grown in Central and South America, Australia, and the United States. The tiny seeds have huge nutritional benefits, containing significant amounts of vitamins and minerals including B vitamins, folate, calcium, iron, magnesium, manganese, phosphorus, and zinc, as well as a higher protein content than most plants. The ancient Aztecs and Mayans who grew the *Salvia hispanica* plant understood the value of its seeds, trading them as a major commodity and using them for both culinary and medicinal benefits.

In ancient times, chia was used as a medicinal remedy for everything from digestive issues to infections. But after Spanish colonization of Mesoamerica began, the cultivation of the plant dropped dramatically. Today, however, chia seeds are enjoying a renaissance, becoming recognizable worldwide as a superfood. The excellent nutritional profile of chia seeds makes them a great addition to any diet, but there is also evidence that suggests the seeds provide more than just a dietary boost.

Health Benefits

Some believe that the hydrophilic nature of the seeds can promote weight loss, by expanding in the stomach and preventing overeating; while there is no real evidence to back up this claim, it certainly doesn't hurt to add the power-packed seeds to your daily diet. In fact, there is evidence that chia seeds can help lower both blood pressure and blood sugar, preventing heart disease and diabetes. Chia has also been proven to be an effective performance enhancer when consumed in a beverage during vigorous exercise, without the sugar usually found in sports drinks like Gatorade. Topically, the oil extracted from chia seeds has its own list of benefits, providing relief from chronically itchy and dry skin.

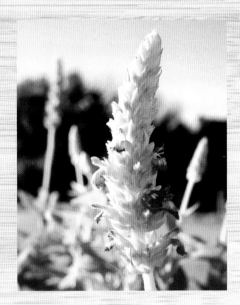

Ideas for Use

Chia seeds are extremely easy to find and to incorporate into your diet. The little black seeds, which have a mild, nutty flavor, are found in most grocery stores and can be consumed raw, sprinkled on oatmeal, cereal, or yogurt, or blended into smoothies. The seeds are also an ingredient in many breads, energy bars, granolas, and even beverages. To use the seeds as an egg substitute, simply mix one tablespoon of chia seeds with three tablespoons of water for each egg in a recipe. Let the mixture sit for 10 to 15 minutes until a gel forms, then add to your recipe.

Cautions

Because the seeds expand when they encounter liquid, it's best to avoid eating them on their own and instead mix them with other foods or liquids first. In rare cases, large amounts of dry seeds can cause blockages in the digestive system, especially in people with a history of swallowing difficulties. For the same reasons, be sure the keep chia seeds away from small children.

Celery Seed

Celery is a staple in many kitchens around the world. It's perfect for creating soup stock, dipping into blue cheese dressing alongside Buffalo wings, or simply eating plain as a crunchy snack. But there's more to this familiar vegetable than its long, fibrous stalks and green, leafy stems. In fact, the tiniest part of this plant may hold the biggest benefits.

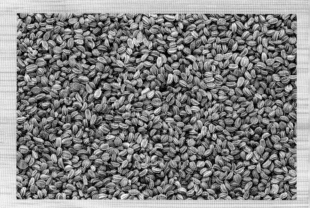

History

Celery has been grown since ancient times, probably originating somewhere in the Mediterranean region, where the vegetable thrived in marshy soils. As it became more popular in less temperate regions, celery was grown as a winter vegetable, and was considered a healing tonic that could provide extra nutrients in seasons when other vegetables were scarce. Today, different varieties of the vegetable—including Pascal celery, popular in North America; celery root, popular in Europe; and leaf celery, popular in Asia—are grown year-round and can easily be purchased at any grocery store.

Good Seeds

Although its culinary uses are obvious in modern times, the vegetable was used mostly for medicinal reasons when it was first cultivated. And while the stalks and leaves have been found to contain their fair share of health benefits, it is the seeds of celery, which are actually very small fruits, that deserve a more visible place in the kitchen—and maybe also the medicine cabinet.

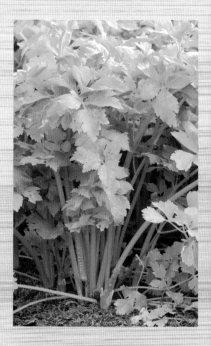

They may be small, but a tablespoon of celery seeds contains large amounts of important nutrients, including 12 percent of the daily intake of calcium, 17 percent of iron, and 27 percent of manganese—all for just 25 calories. Celery seed's high concentration of calcium and manganese help to support and create bone tissue and cartilage, crucial for preventing bone loss, fractures, and osteoporosis, especially in older adults.

Mineral Benefits

The iron content in celery seed is also a boon to health, helping the body produce red blood cells and stave off anemia. The iron in the seeds is "non-heme" iron, which is different than the "heme" iron found in animal products. Because this iron is from a plant and not an animal, the body absorbs it at a lower rate. To counteract this effect, be sure to consume celery seeds with foods rich in vitamin C, such as citrus fruits or bell peppers. The vitamin C enhances the absorption of non-heme iron, ensuring the greatest benefit from the tiny seeds.

Celery seed is also a great source of magnesium, with one tablespoon providing around 10 percent of daily intake. This mineral plays an important role in the regulation of blood sugar, helping to increase cells' response to insulin, and studies have shown that magnesium-rich diets reduce the risk of type 2 diabetes by 14 percent.

Help for the Heart?

The nutritional profile of celery seed is only the beginning of its benefits. The seeds have also been prized since antiquity in Ayurvedic medicine for their effect on the cardiovascular system. Celery seeds are a natural diuretic, helping to speed the excretion of salt from the body. Since excess salt can cause a fluid buildup in the blood vessels and cause high blood pressure, celery seeds are a natural way to lower blood pressure. A 2013 study published in the *Journal of Medicinal Food* demonstrated that the seed lowered blood pressure in animals with high blood pressure, while having no effect on those with normal blood pressure.

Other Health Benefits

Celery seed has also been found to have anti-inflammatory, antioxidant, and possibly antibacterial properties, helping to relieve the pain of arthritis, reduce muscle cramps, and prevent infections. There have even been studies that indicate celery seed extract can prevent the spread of liver cancer and stomach cancer, although more research is needed to uncover the extent of its cancer-fighting properties.

Ideas for Use

Celery seed smells and tastes just like the vegetable itself, and can be found as whole seeds, crushed, or ground up. The seeds can be added to salads, used in spice rubs, mixed into casseroles, or used in pickling recipes, and the ground spice is sometimes used as a salt substitute. The seed can also be found in supplement form, which can be taken to help with blood pressure regulation or to prevent urinary tract infections. Be sure to check with a doctor to find a dosage that is appropriate for your condition.

Cinnamon

Zeylanicum or "true" cinnamon starts off as the dry inner bark of a large 20-to-30-foot tree most likely growing in Sri Lanka. The Arabs, Portuguese, Dutch, and British successively controlled trade of this valuable spice. Then, as now, cinnamon flavored mouthwashes, foods, and drinks, and was used as an aphrodisiac. Cinnamon's scent also stirs the appetite, invigorates and "warms" the senses, and may even produce a feeling of joy. There are two main kinds of essential oil made from zeylanicum. The oil made from the bark is the most pungently cinnamonlike, while a milder oil is made from the leaves.

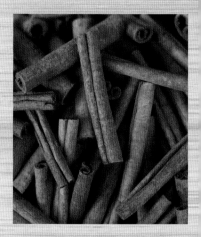

Native to China, cassia is sometimes called "Chinese cinnamon," and is very similar to "true" cinnamon. But cassia is actually the most common kind of cinnamon sold in the United States. The dried bark of this evergreen tree has the familiar spicy scent so ubiquitous in a multitude of food and drinks throughout the world. But beyond its obvious worth as a flavoring agent, cassia essential oil has been employed medicinally as far back as biblical times. And in traditional Chinese medicine, the spice is considered one of the 50 fundamental herbs in the practice.

Health Benefits

In general, cinnamon is used as a physical and emotional stimulant. Researchers have found that it reduces drowsiness, irritability, and the pain and number of headaches. In one study, the aroma of cinnamon in the room helped participants to concentrate and perform better. The essential oil and its fragrance help relax tight muscles, ease painful joints, and relieve menstrual cramps.

Cassia has antibacterial properties that can prevent infections in minor cuts or scrapes. In its essential oil form, it is a warming oil, which makes it excellent for improving circulation and relieving pain caused by arthritis or sore muscles. The oil has been used for centuries as a cure for diarrhea and to promote healthy digestion. Cassia can be used to repel insects—especially as a mosquito repellent. Many studies have suggested that cassia can help lower blood sugar, making it a good oil to have on hand for diabetics. Because of its warming properties, cassia can irritate the skin or cause allergic reactions. It's best to do a patch test before using. Ingesting too much of the oil can be harmful to the liver, so always use in minute amounts. Since it may lower blood sugar, diabetics who are on medication should be sure to closely monitor blood sugar to be sure it doesn't dip too low.

Folk Remedies

Cure cold feet with some nice hot cinnamon tea. Stir a gram of powdered cinnamon into a glass of hot water and steep for 15 minutes. Drink three times a day.

Good sleep habits are important in the treatment of PMS, and a brew of cinnamon tea is relaxing just before bed. Sweeten to taste with honey.

Cinnamon has anti-inflammatory and antispasmodic properties that relieve menstrual cramps. Use as a tea, or sprinkle on toast or sweet rolls. If you have a heavy period, drinking cinnamon tea the day before or during your period may help.

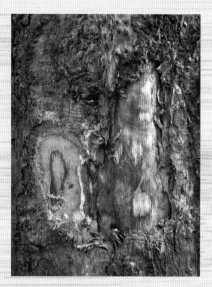

This is a traditional remedy for acid relief. Brew a cup of cinnamon tea from a cinnamon stick. Or try a commercial brand, but check the label. Cinnamon tea often has black tea in it, which is a cause of heartburn, so make sure your commercial brand doesn't contain black tea. For another acid-busting treat, make cinnamon toast.

Eat pumpkin baked as a squash to get rid of heartburn. Fresh is best. Spice it up with cinnamon, or, make a compote of baked pumpkin and apples, spiced with cinnamon and honey, for a dessert that's both curative and tasty.

For a sore throat, mix 2 parts cinnamon, 2 parts ginger, and 3 parts licorice powder. Steep 1 teaspoon of this mixture in 1 cup boiling water for ten minutes, then drink as a sore throat cure three times a day.

Holiday Blend

Instead of burning sooty candles or spraying air fresheners full of chemicals, try a festive blend of essential oils this holiday season. This bright and spicy mix will fill your home with holiday warmth and cheer, without the unwanted toxins.

- 3 drops cinnamon oil
- 3 drops orange oil
- 2 drops clove oil
- 1 drop cardamom oil
- 1 drop ginger oil

Combine all essential oils and add to a diffuser.

Note that cinnamon, clove, and ginger essential oils are all known dermal irritants, so be careful while handling them.

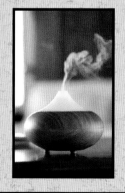

Good Morning Bread

- 1 cup mashed ripe bananas (about 3 medium)
- ¼ cup warm milk (130°F)
- 3 tablespoons vegetable or canola oil
- 2¼ cups bread flour, divided
- ¾ cup whole wheat flour
- ½ cup old-fashioned oats
- 1 package (¼ ounce) rapid-rise active dry yeast
- 1 teaspoon salt
- 1 teaspoon grated orange peel
- 1 teaspoon ground cinnamon

1. Combine bananas, milk and oil in medium bowl; mix well. Whisk ½ cup bread flour, whole wheat flour, oats, yeast, salt, orange peel and cinnamon in large bowl of electric stand mixer. Add banana mixture; beat at medium speed 3 minutes with paddle attachment.

2. Replace paddle attachment with dough hook; beat in enough remaining bread flour to form soft dough. Knead at medium-low speed 5 minutes or until dough is smooth and elastic. Place dough in greased bowl; turn dough so top is greased. Cover and let rise in warm place about 30 minutes or until doubled in size. (Dense loaf might not double in size.)

3. Spray 9X5-inch loaf pan with nonstick cooking spray. Punch down dough; shape into loaf. Place in prepared pan; cover and let rise in warm place about 30 minutes or until doubled in size. Preheat oven to 375°F.

4. Bake about 35 minutes or until browned and loaf sounds hollow when tapped/internal temperature reaches 200°F. Remove to wire rack to cool completely.

Makes 1 loaf

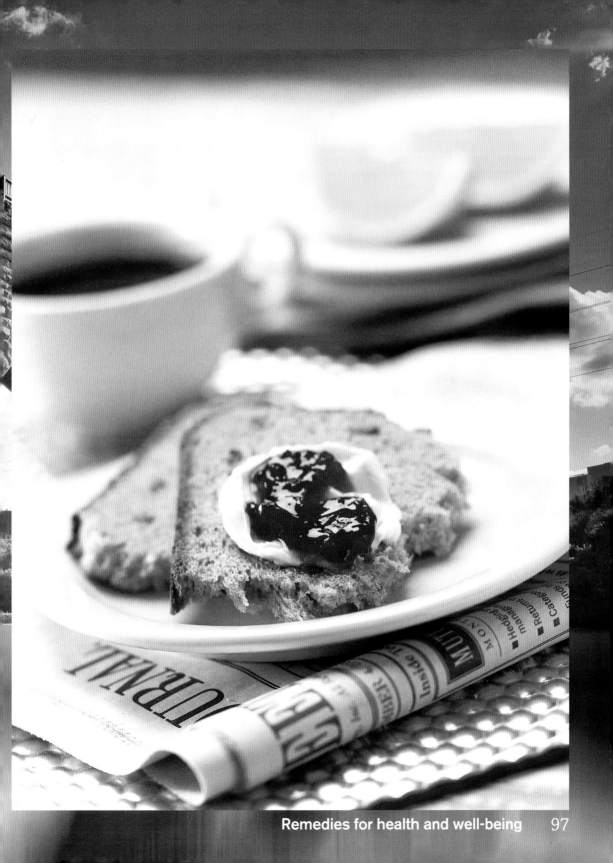

Cloves

In ancient China, courtiers at the Han court held cloves in their mouths to freshen their breath before they had an audience with the emperor. Today, cloves are still used to sweeten breath. Modern dental preparations numb tooth and gum pain and quell infection with clove essential oil or its main constituent, eugenol. The familiar clove buds used to poke hams and flavor mulled wine are picked while still unripe and dried before being shipped or distilled into essential oil.

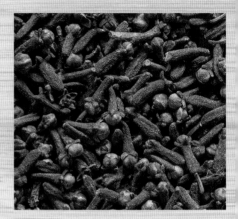

History

Simply inhaling the fragrance of cloves was once said to improve eyesight and fend off the plague. Clove's scent developed a reputation, now backed by science, for being stimulating. The fragrance was also believed to be an aphrodisiac. Cloves were so valuable that a Frenchman risked his life to steal a clove tree from the Dutch colonies in Indonesia and plant it in French ground. Once established, the slender evergreen trees bear buds for at least a century.

Use as an Essential Oil

As an antiseptic and pain reliever, clove essential oil relieves toothaches, flu, colds, and bronchial congestion. But don't try to use it straight on an infant's gums for teething as is often suggested, or you may end up with a screaming baby because it tastes so strong and hot. Instead mix only two drops of clove oil in at least a teaspoon of vegetable oil. It can still be hot, however, so try it in your own mouth first. Then apply it directly to the baby's gums.

In a heating liniment, clove essential oil helps sore muscles and arthritis. Mix 30 drops of clove essential oil in one ounce of apple cider vinegar, shake well, and dab on athlete's foot.

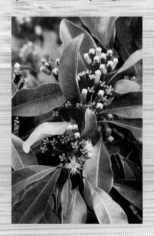

Researchers have found that the spicy aroma of clove reduces drowsiness, irritability, and headaches.

Precaution: The essential oil irritates skin and mucous membranes, so be sure to dilute it before use. Clove leaf is almost pure eugenol; do not use it in aromatherapy preparations.

A Happy Mouth

Chewing on the seeds of aromatic spices such as clove, cardamom, or fennel after meals is a common practice in South Asia and the Middle East. The seeds of these spices contain antimicrobial properties that can help halt bad breath.

Ground cloves have been used to relieve toothaches for thousands of years. Moisten 1 teaspoon powdered cloves in olive oil and pack it into an aching cavity. Dentists still use a mixture of eugenol and zinc oxide before applying amalgam when filling teeth.

To relieve denture discomfort, blend 1 teaspoon cloves into a powder using a coffee grinder or use ½ teaspoon prepackaged ground cloves. Moisten with olive oil and dab around a mouth or gum sore.

Ideas for Use

Cloves are reputed to pep up digestion and eliminate gas. Add 2 to 3 whole cloves to rice before cooking. Sprinkle on apples and pears when baking. Or steep 2 to 3 whole cloves in a cup of boiling water for ten minutes, sweeten to taste, and drink.

When you have a sore throat, try this Russian sore throat cure. Combine 1 tablespoon pure horseradish or horseradish root with 1 teaspoon honey and 1 teaspoon ground cloves. Mix in a glass of warm water and drink slowly.

Clove also makes a nice nausea-fighting tea. Brew a cup using 1 teaspoon clove powder in a teacup full of boiling water. Strain out any clove that might be remaining, and drink as needed.

Essential Oil

Immunity Boosting Diffusion Blend

- 3 drops clove oil
- 3 drops lemon oil
- 2 drops cinnamon oil
- 2 drops eucalyptus oil
- 1 drop rosemary oil
- Water

Fill diffuser with as much water as needed and add the oils. Turn diffuser on in a central location for maximum effect.

Note that cinnamon and clove essential oils are known dermal irritants.

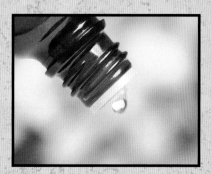

Mulled Cranberry Tea

- 2 black tea bags
- 1 cup boiling water
- 1 bottle (48 ounces) cranberry juice
- ½ cup dried cranberries (optional)
- ⅓ cup sugar
- 1 large lemon, cut into 1/4-inch slices
- 4 cinnamon sticks
- 6 whole cloves

***Additional thin lemon slices and cinnamon sticks (optional)

1. Place tea bags in slow cooker. Pour boiling water over tea bags; cover and let stand 5 minutes. Remove and discard tea bags. Stir in cranberry juice, cranberries, if desired, sugar, lemon slices, 4 cinnamon sticks and cloves. Cover; cook on LOW 2 to 3 hours or on HIGH 1 to 2 hours.

2. Remove and discard lemon slices, cinnamon sticks and cloves. Serve in warm mugs with additional lemon slices and cinnamon sticks, if desired.

Makes 8 servings

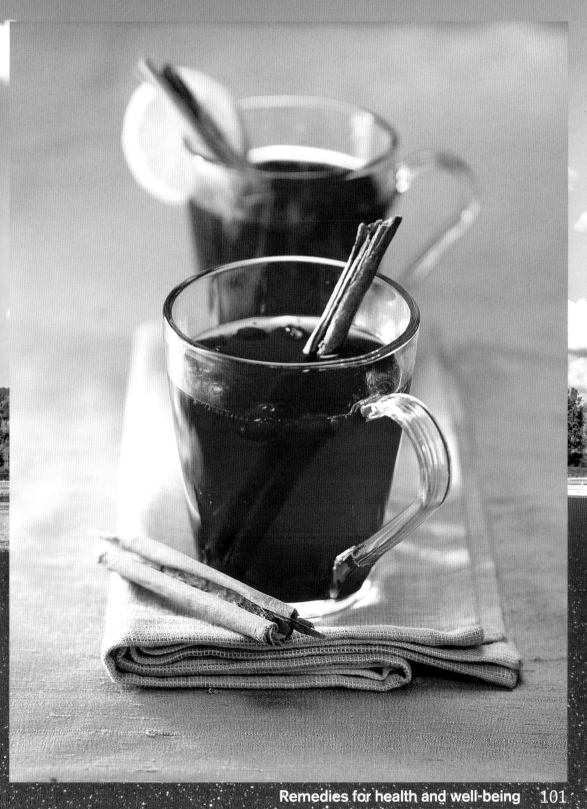

Coriander

The coriander plant is synonymous with cilantro. Generally, the fresh plant is called cilantro, while the seeds are referred to as coriander. This plant native to west Asia, Europe, and the eastern Mediterranean has been used for centuries as an aphrodisiac, to lift spirits, assist digestion, and restore calm. The seeds were reputedly found in the tomb of the Egyptian pharaoh Rameses II. It is widely cultivated in Morocco, Mexico, Argentina, Canada, India, and the United States, especially in South Carolina.

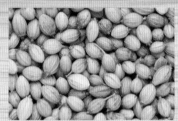

Coriander's leaf flavor is a cross between sage and citrus. The herb's bold flavor is common to several ethnic cuisines, notably those of China, southeast Asia, Mexico, East India, Spain, Central Africa, and Central and South America.

Growing the Plant

Coriander's bright green, lacy leaves resemble those of flat-leaved Italian parsley when they first spring up from seed, but they become more fernlike as the plant matures. Coriander flowers from middle to late summer. The herb is native to the eastern Mediterranean region and southern Europe. Coriander prefers average, well-drained soil in full sun.

A Long History

Coriander has been cultivated for 3,000 years. The Hebrews, who used coriander seed as one of their Passover herbs, probably learned about it from the ancient Egyptians, who revered the plant. The Romans and Greeks used coriander for medicinal purposes and as a spice and preservative. The Chinese believed coriander could make a human immortal. Throughout northern Europe, people would suck on candy-coated coriander seeds when they had indigestion.

Make Your Own Deodorant

The most important action of any deodorant is to kill bacteria, which essential oils do very well. By making your own deodorant, you can soothe rashes and irritations and avoid the use of the harsh, pore-blocking ingredients found in commercial products.

15 drops lavender oil

5 drops sage oil

5 drops coriander oil

2 ounces aloe vera juice or witch hazel

Combine all ingredients in a spray bottle. Shake well before each use. This will keep at least a year.

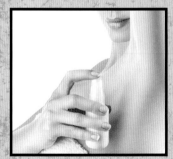

Remedies and Benefits

Chewing the seeds soothes an upset stomach, relieves flatulence, aids digestion, and improves appetite. Poultices of coriander seeds have been used to relieve the pain of rheumatism. The Chinese prescribe the tea to treat dysentery and measles. Coriander relieves inflammation and headaches. But its most popular medicinal use has been to flavor strong-tasting medicines and to prevent intestinal gripping common with some laxative formulas.

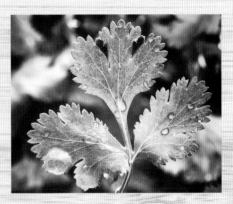

When you're having dental problems, this spice, as well as thyme and green tea, has antibacterial properties. Brew a tea from your choice of the three and use as a mouth rinse after meals.

When suffering from flatulence, crush the seeds into powder and add to foods such as vegetable stir-fry.

Ideas for Use

Add young leaves to beets, onions, salads, sausage, clams, oysters, and potatoes. Add seeds to marinades, salad dressings, cheese, eggs, and pickling brines. Coriander seed is used commercially to flavor sugared confections, liqueurs such as Benedictine and Chartreuse, and gin. Its flavor really enhances curry and Middle Eastern dishes, too.

Very large doses are reputedly narcotic, but it is unlikely you could eat the quantity needed to produce this effect.

The Essential Oil

The essential oil of coriander is not distilled from the herb, but rather from the seeds. It has a pungent and refreshing aroma, with sweet and slightly woody and peppery overtones. Aromatherapists attribute to it he ability to quell bad moods, calm frayed nerves, and promote feelings of relaxation. The essential oil is found in perfumes, aftershaves, and cosmetics because of its delightfully spicy scent. It is no longer as popular a cosmetic as it was from the 14th to 17th centuries, but coriander "refines" the complexion and was in the famous Eau de Carnes and Carmelite water. It is still used in soaps and deodorants.

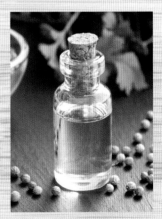

Quinoa Pancakes with Tomato Chutney

Tomato Chutney

- 1 tablespoon vegetable oil
- ½ teaspoon cumin seeds
- ½ onion, finely chopped
- 2 cloves garlic, finely chopped
- 2 teaspoons grated fresh ginger
- 2 cups tomatoes, seeded and chopped
- 1 green chile, seeded and chopped (optional)
- 1 teaspoon ground coriander
- 1 teaspoon salt
- 2 teaspoons sugar

Pancakes

- 1 cup buttermilk pancake mix
- 1 cup red quinoa, cooked and cooled
- 1 egg, beaten
- 1¼ cups fat-free (skim) milk
- 1 cup spinach, finely chopped

1. For chutney, heat oil in small skillet over medium heat. Add cumin seeds; cook several seconds until seeds stop popping. Add onion, garlic and ginger; cook and stir 1 to 2 minutes or until onions are translucent. Add tomatoes, green chile, coriander and salt; cook 3 to 4 minutes until tomatoes are soft, stirring occasionally. Stir in sugar. Set aside to cool 5 to 10 minutes.

2. Add chutney to blender or food processor; pulse until chutney has uniformly coarse texture. Serve immediately or cover and refrigerate. (Chutney will keep in refrigerator up to 1 week.)

3. For pancakes, combine pancake mix and quinoa in medium bowl; mix well. Stir in egg and milk until blended. Fold in spinach. Let stand 10 minutes.

4. Spray medium skillet with nonstick cooking spray; heat over medium heat. Pour ¼ cup batter into skillet for each pancake; cook until tops are bubbled and the bottoms are lightly browned. Turn pancakes; cook 1 minute. Serve warm with Tomato Chutney.

Makes 5 servings

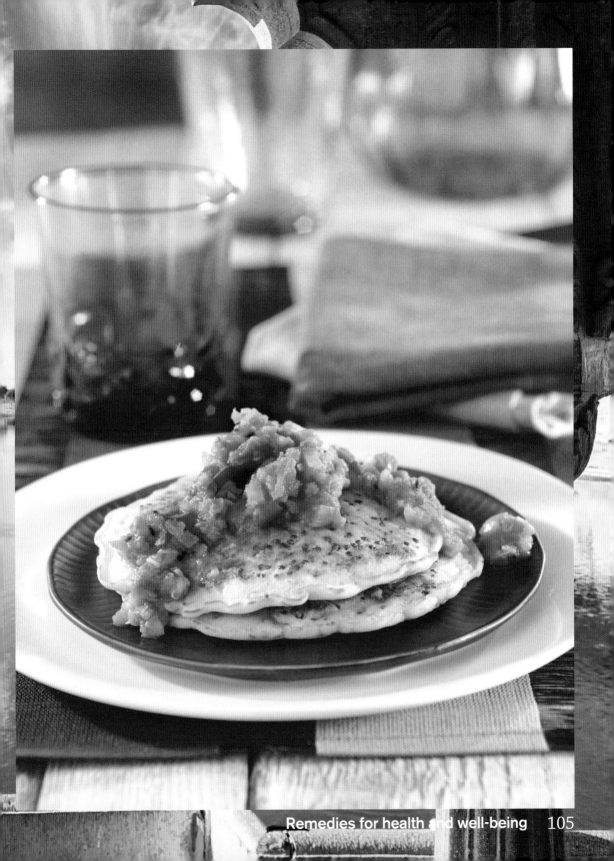

Cumin

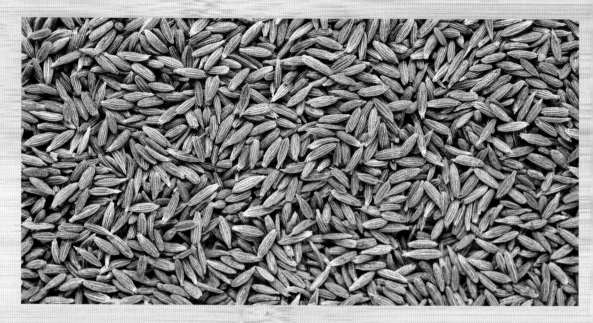

The plant that provides cumin seeds is a member of the parsley family that probably originated thousands of years ago in the Mediterranean region. It was known to the ancient Egyptians and even used in the mummification process; it's still used today in Egypt in the versatile dip called Duqqa or Dukkah. An essential component of curry powder, cumin is very popular in Indian food, as well as adding flavor Mexican foods and Middle Eastern dishes. Cumin is related to caraway, and their seeds are similar in appearance and have many of the same anti-indigestion properties.

A Loving Spice?

In the Middle Ages, wives sent their soldier husbands off to war with a loaf of cumin bread, symbolizing love. A combination of cumin, black pepper, and honey was believed to have aphrodisiac qualities, although there is, fortunately or unfortunately, no evidence to back up this use.

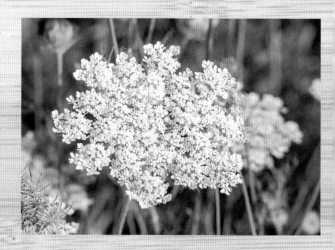

Folk Remedies

For swollen feet, mix ¼ teaspoon each of cumin, coriander, and fennel into a cup of hot water and drink two to three times a day.

To relieve belching, roast equal amounts of cumin, fennel, and celery seed. Combine. After you eat, chew well about ½ to 1 teaspoon of the mixture, then chase it down with ⅓ cup of warm water.

Steep a tea with 1 teaspoon cumin seeds and a pinch of nutmeg to soothe tummy troubles.

To relieve PMS symptoms such as backache and abdominal pain, add a pinch of cumin to 1 tablespoon aloe vera gel, and take three times a day with meals.

Health Benefits

Cumin seeds are a good source of iron and other essential minerals such as manganese, copper, magnesium, and calcium. Cumin has been used medicinally in a number of medical traditions, including Ayurvedic medicine, often for indigestion. One small 2013 study of people suffering from irritable bowel syndrome found that cumin essential oil could help relieve symptoms such as abdominal pain and nausea. Some research has been done on the use of cumin to help people lose weight, control high cholesterol, and control blood sugar levels in those suffereing from diabetes; study results have varied. Cumin also contains some anti-inflammatory compounds, although there have not been sufficient studies to determine whether cumin can help reduce inflammation in people. It may have diuretic properties, so people take it to relieve bloating; again, concrete evidence is scant.

Ideas for Use

Cumin pairs well with legumes, rice, and vegetables. Paired with coriander and sometimes other herbs or spices, it's part of the Indian spice mix known as Dhana jiru.

Cautions

While cumin is generally considered safe in food, diabetes should be careful of taking large amounts since blood sugar might lower.

Cumin Confusion

Note that black cumin seed oil, an essential oil, comes from the plant *Nigella sativa*, also called black caraway, black seed, or the fennel flower. Cumin comes from the *Cuminum cyminum* plant.

Curry Beef

- 1 pound 90% lean ground beef
- 1 medium onion, thinly sliced
- ½ cup beef broth
- 1 tablespoon curry powder
- 1 teaspoon ground cumin
- 2 cloves garlic, minced
- 1 cup sour cream
- ¼ cup reduced-fat (2%) milk
- ½ cup raisins, divided
- 1 teaspoon sugar
- 12 ounces uncooked wide egg noodles or 1⅓ cups uncooked long grain white rice
- ¼ cup chopped walnuts, almonds or pecans

1. Brown beef 6 to 8 minutes in large skillet over medium-high heat, stirring to break up meat. Drain fat. Combine beef, onion, broth, curry powder, cumin and garlic in slow cooker. Cover; cook on LOW 4 hours.

2. Stir in sour cream, milk, ¼ cup raisins and sugar. Cover; cook 30 minutes or until thickened and heated through.

3. Cook noodles according to package directions; drain. Spoon beef curry over noodles. Sprinkle with remaining ¼ cup raisins and walnuts.

Makes 4 servings

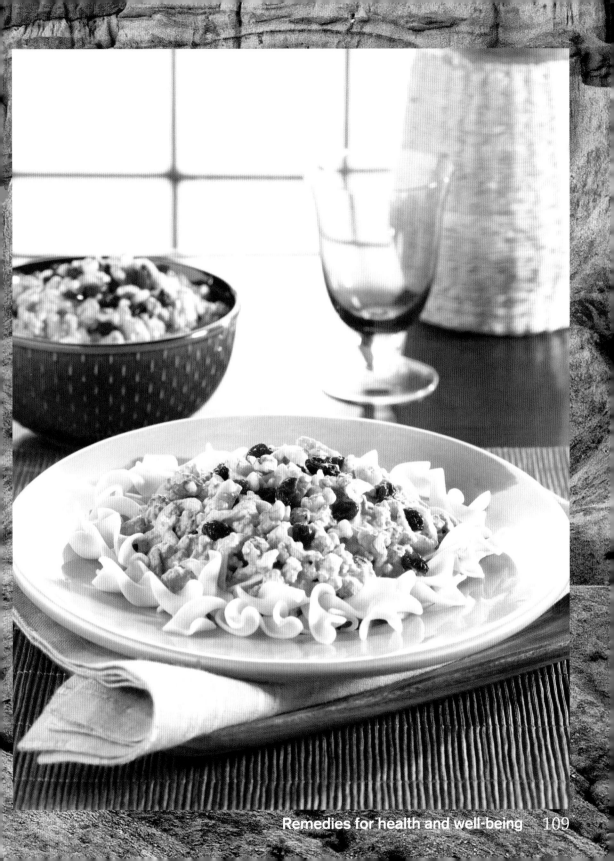

Dill Seed

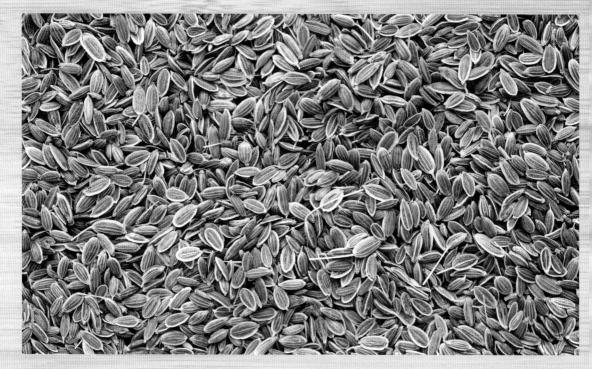

Dill's obvious claim to fame is its inclusion in pickle recipes. What deli sandwich would be complete without a dill pickle on the side? The biennial herb was called *Anethon* by the ancient Egyptians, Greeks, and Romans—its botanical name was derived from this word. Our word comes from the Old English *dylle*, which means "to lull." A fitting description, as dill essential oil is known to have soothing, calming properties. In fact, Romans used to rub themselves with dill oil before heading into battle, to calm their nerves!

Traditional Medicine

Dill derives from an old Norse word meaning "to lull," and, indeed, the herb once was used to induce sleep in babies with colic. Herbalists also use dill to relieve gas and to stimulate flow of mother's milk. Dill stimulates the appetite and settles the stomach, but the seeds have also been chewed to lessen the appetite and stop the stomach from rumbling—something that parishioners found useful during all-day church services.

In India, it is used to treat ulcers, fevers, uterine pain, and problems with the eyes and kidneys, usually in a formula with other herbs. In Ethiopia, the seeds are chewed to relieve a headache.

To relieve belching, drop 1 teaspoon dill seeds into 1 cup boiling water, then steep for 15 minutes. Strain, then drink.

Swallowing a teaspoon of dill seeds is an old folk remedy for hiccups that may work for you. No one is sure if it's an ingredient in the dill seeds that helps or if simply swallowing the seeds is what does the trick.

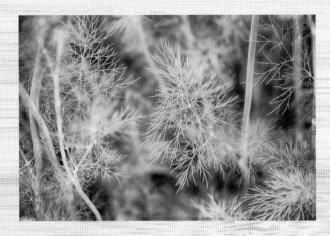

Though scientists haven't proved its worth, dill seed is often used as a folk cure for insomnia in China. Its essential oil has the most sedative-producing properties.

Ideas for Use

Add minced dill leaves to salads and use as a garnish. Seeds go well with fish, lamb, pork, poultry, cheese, cream, eggs, and an array of vegetables, including cabbage, onions, cauliflower, squash, spinach, potatoes, and broccoli. Of course, dill pickles would not be the same without dill seed and weed. The herb is particularly popular in Russia and Scandinavia. Its taste somewhat resembles caraway, which shares a similar chemistry.

By far, the most popular way to use dill is to incorporate it into your food to aid digestion. Although you could use it in an herb tea, sweeter digestive herbs such as anise are preferred.

Dill Essential Oil

Dill oil can help prevent infections, both internal and external, and can even prevent lice infestations if applied to the scalp. The oil can relieve muscle spasms and calm cramps. It has been used for millennia as a way to support healthy digestion, and helps alleviate constipation, gas, and indigestion. When used in aromatherapy, its calming, sedative properties help relieve anxiety and promote a good night's sleep.

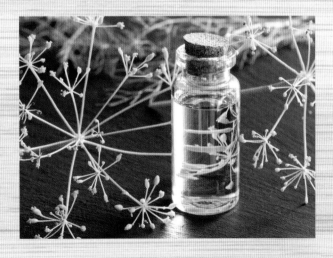

Dilly Deviled Eggs

- 6 hard-cooked eggs, peeled and cut in half lengthwise
- 2 tablespoons plain low-fat Greek yogurt
- 1 tablespoon light mayonnaise
- 1 tablespoon minced fresh dill or 1 teaspoon dried dill weed
- 1 tablespoon minced dill pickle
- 1 teaspoon Dijon mustard
- $1/8$ teaspoon salt
- $1/8$ teaspoon white pepper

***Paprika (optional)
***Dill sprigs (optional)

1. Remove yolks from egg halves. Mash yolks with yogurt, yogurt, dill, pickle, mustard, salt and pepper in small bowl.

2. Fill egg halves with mixture using teaspoon or piping bag fitted with large plain tip. Garnish with paprika and dill sprigs.

Makes 8 servings

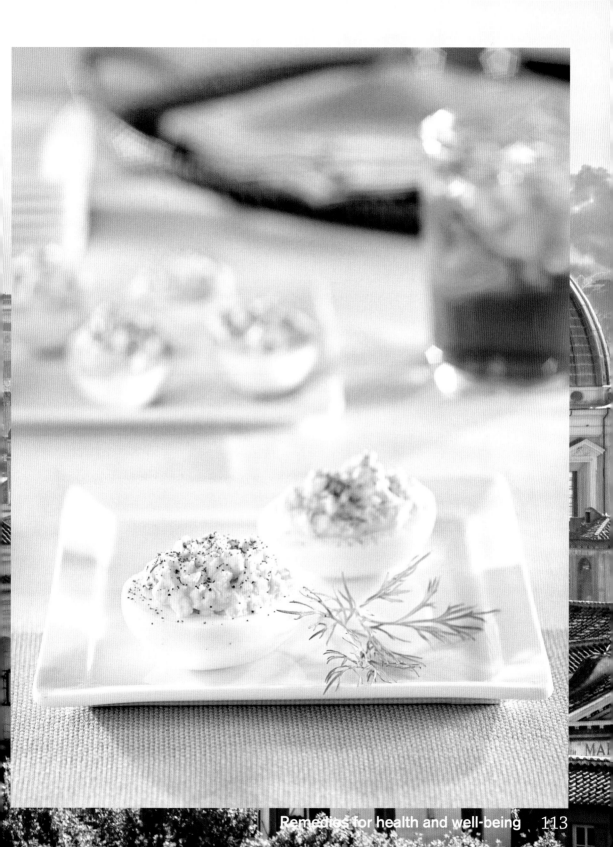

Fennel

Known for its licorice-like flavor, fennel, a member of the carrot family, is native to the Mediterranean. But the flowering plant is now found all over the world, including Europe and the United States, and is coveted for both its taste and its therapeutic benefits. The herb was noted for its medicinal properties as far back as the 10th century, and even the poet Henry Wadsworth Longfellow wrote about fennel's "wondrous powers." Today, the herb is commonly used in foods, drinks, and cosmetics, but it is especially prized for its effectiveness at treating digestive issues.

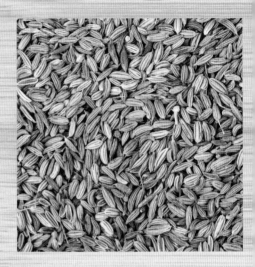

Traditional Medical Uses

The Greeks gave fennel to nursing mothers to increase milk flow. Early physicians also considered fennel a remedy for poor eyesight, weight loss, hiccups, nausea, gout, and many other illnesses. Fennel is a carminative (relieves gas and pain in the bowels), weak diuretic, and mild digestive stimulant. Herbalists often recommend fennel tea to soothe an upset stomach and dispel gas. It aids digestion, especially of fat.

In Europe, a popular children's carminative is still made with fennel, chamomile, caraway, coriander, and bitter orange peel.

Fennel is also a urinary tract tonic that lessens inflammation and helps eliminate kidney stones.

For swollen feet, mix ¼ teaspoon each of cumin, coriander, and fennel into a cup of hot water and drink two to three times a day.

To relieve belching, roast equal amounts of cumin, fennel, and celery seed. Combine. After you eat, chew well about ½ to 1 teaspoon of the mixture, then chase it down with ⅓ cup of warm water.

Chewing on fennel seeds after meals is a common practice in South Asia and the Middle East. The seeds contain antimicrobial properties that can help halt bad breath.

Munching on fennel seeds mixed with aniseed can help combat bad breath that accompanies dry mouth. In addition, fennel seed can be combined with other herbs to make a mouthwash.

To relieve gas, drink it as a tea by steeping ½ teaspoon seeds in 1 cup boiling water for ten minutes. Or, sprinkle them over those gassy vegetables during cooking or add to stir-fries. If you've acquired the taste, fennel also works well cooked into figs, apples, pears, and plums.

Fennel, like its cousin caraway, is a familiar digestive aid for boosting the appetite.

Fennel seeds may be able to relieve the intestinal spasms associated with IBS. They may also aid in the elimination of fats from the digestive system, inhibiting the over-production of mucus in the intestine, which is a symptom of the ailment. Steep the seeds into a tea by adding ½ teaspoon fennel to 1 cup boiling water. Or add them to veggies such as carrots or cabbage, both of which soothe IBS symptoms. You can also sprinkle the seeds on salads or roast them and snack on them after a meal to reduce the symptoms of IBS and freshen your breath. To roast, spritz a baking sheet with olive oil, then cover with fennel seeds. Bake at 325°F for 10 to 15 minutes.

Ideas for Use

Fennel tastes like a more bitter version of anise. Use leaves in salads and as garnishes. You can eat tender stems as you would celery, and add seeds to desserts, breads, cakes, cookies, and beverages. Mince bulbs of sweet fennel and eat raw or braise. Fennel complements fish, sausage, duck, barley, rice, cabbage, beets, pickles, potatoes, lentils, breads, and eggs. Add it to butters, cheese spreads, and salad dressings.

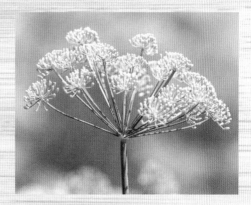

Fennel Essential Oil

Fennel essential oil is found commercially in condiments, liqueurs, and aromatherapy cosmetics such as creams, perfumes, and soaps. It has a reputation for improving the complexion and decreasing wrinkles.

Cautions

Fennel has mild estrogenic properties, so avoid it if you're pregnant. Very large amounts can overstimulate the nervous system. Be especially careful using the essential oil.

Fresh Tomato Pasta Soup

- 1 tablespoon olive oil
- ½ cup chopped onion
- 1 clove garlic, minced
- 3 pounds fresh tomatoes (about 9 medium), coarsely chopped
- 3 cups fat-free reduced-sodium chicken broth
- 1 tablespoon minced fresh basil
- 1 tablespoon minced fresh marjoram
- 1 tablespoon minced fresh oregano
- 1 teaspoon whole fennel seeds
- ½ teaspoon black pepper
- ¾ cup uncooked rosamarina, orzo or other small pasta
- ½ cup (2 ounces) shredded part-skim mozzarella cheese

1. Heat oil in large saucepan over medium heat. Add onion and garlic; cook and stir until onion is tender.

2. Add tomatoes, broth, basil, marjoram, oregano, fennel seeds and pepper; bring to a boil. Reduce heat to low; cover and simmer 25 minutes. Remove from heat; cool slightly.

3. Purée tomato mixture in batches in food processor or blender. Return to saucepan; bring to a boil. Add pasta; cook 7 to 9 minutes or until tender. Sprinkle with cheese.

Makes 8 servings

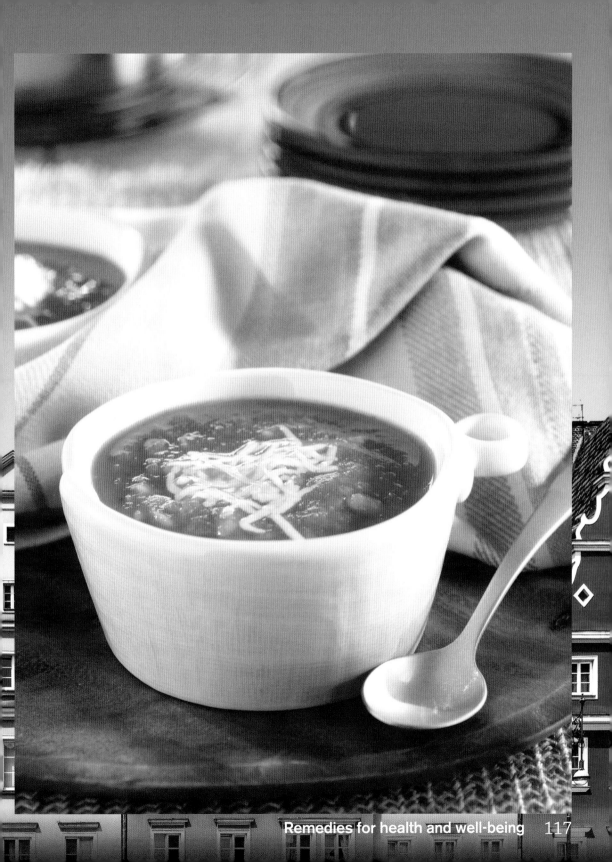

Garlic

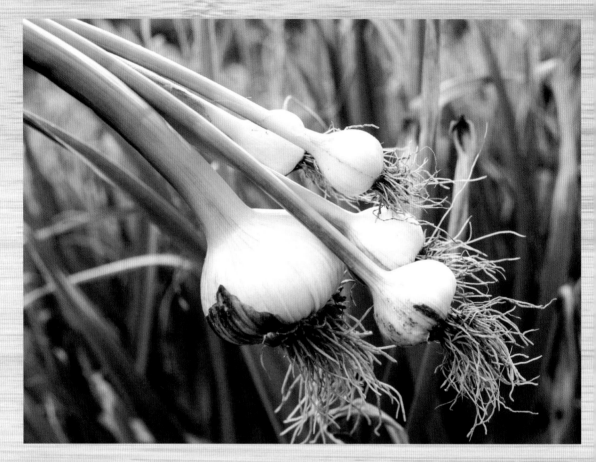

The wonders of garlic have been with us for millennia. Writings from ancient Egypt, Greece, India, and China all make mention of the humble garlic clove. It has long been used in many cultures to improve health or to transform meals into delicious, aromatic delights. Its ability to enhance flavor is undeniable, while the extent of its healing benefits continues to be revealed.

Garlic, or scientifically speaking, *Allium sativum*, is cultivated across the globe, except in the polar regions. The bulb of this attractive plant contains more powerful sulfur compounds than does any other Allium species, such as onions and leeks. The garlic plant may have evolved to include these smelly sulfur compounds as a way of warding off foraging animals, invasive insects, and even soil-borne microorganisms such as bacteria and fungi. Yet these same compounds, which lend garlic its pungent aroma and delectable flavor as well as its medicinal qualities, are exactly the reason so many people are attracted to the bulb.

Garlic Varieties

There are actually more than 400 species and varieties of garlic. *Allium sativum* is the most common type of garlic; it is the one you'll typically find in the grocery store and is often called "culinary" garlic. Fortunately, this is the species that also offers the most healing properties.

You might occasionally find *Allium ursinum* in specialty or farmers' markets. *Allium ursinum* is a type of wild garlic native to Northern Europe that does not possess the same healing properties as *Allium sativum*. You might also come across *Allium vineale*, a garlic with very small cloves that is commonly called "crow garlic." This variety is nothing more than a weed.

Allium sativum has two subvarieties: softneck and hardneck. The two types have similar healing properties because they belong to the same species, but they differ in flavor, clove size, shelf life, and use.

Softneck garlic is the type you'll most likely see in the produce section of your grocery store. Its name comes from the multilayered parchment that covers the entire bulb, continues up the neck of the bulb, and forms a soft, pliable stalk suitable for braiding. Its papery skin, or sheath, is a beautiful creamy white color.

Softneck garlic typically has several layers of cloves surrounding the central portion of the garlic bulb. The outermost layer's cloves are the stoutest; the cloves of the internal layers become smaller closer to the center of the bulb. Of the several types of softneck garlic, two are most abundant:

Silverskin garlic. This easy-to-grow variety has a strong flavor and stores well when dried—it will last nearly a year under the right conditions. The Creole group of silverskin garlics has a rose-tinted parchment.

Artichoke garlic. Artichoke garlic has a milder flavor and may have fewer and larger cloves than silverskin. You can store it as long as eight months. Artichoke garlic may occasionally have purple spots or streaks on its skin, but don't confuse it with purple stripe garlic, a hardneck variety that has quite a bit of purple coloring.

Unlike softneck garlic, hardneck varieties do not have a flexible stalk. When you buy this type of garlic, it will typically have an extremely firm stalk protruding an inch or two from the top of the bulb.

Hardneck garlic sends up scapes from its central woody stalk when it is growing. A scape is a thin green extension of the stalk that forms a 360-degree curl with a small bulbil, or swelling, several inches from its end. Inside the bulbil are more than 100 tiny cloves that are genetically identical to the parent bulb beneath. Many people call these "flowers," but they are not really blooms. If left on the plant, the scape will eventually die and fall over, and the tiny cloves will spill onto the ground. However, most never make it that far.

Cutting off the scapes keeps the plant's energy from forming the bulbil and therefore encourages larger bulbs. But don't throw out the scapes. They can be a delicious ingredient in your cooking. There are three main types of hardneck garlic:

Rocambole. This variety has a rich, full-bodied taste. It peels easily and typically has just one set of cloves around the woody stalk. It keeps for up to six months.

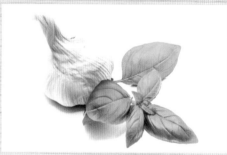

Porcelain. Porcelain garlic is similar to rocambole in flavor and typically contains about four large cloves wrapped in a very smooth, white, papery sheath. People of often mistake porcelain garlic for elephant garlic because its cloves are so large. Porcelain garlic stores well for about eight months.

Purple stripe. This hardneck variety is famous for making the best baked garlic. There are several types of purple stripe, all with distinctive bright purple streaks on their papery sheaths. Purple stripe garlic keeps for about six months.

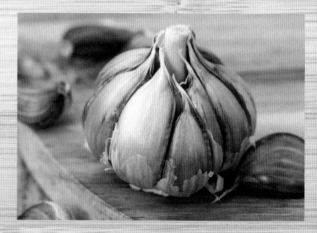

Another member of the Allium clan, elephant garlic (*Allium ampeloprasum*), may look like a good buy because it is so large, but its flavor is very bland. Elephant garlic tastes more like a leek; in fact, its garlic flavor is slight and its healing properties are inferior to those of other garlic varieties. Use elephant garlic more like a vegetable than a flavorful herb.

History

Garlic, which has been grown for more than 5,000 years, is one of the oldest cultivated plants in the world. Researchers think the ancient Egyptians were the first to farm garlic. Ancient Egyptians bestowed many sacred qualities upon garlic. They believed it kept away evil spirits, so they buried garlic-shape lumps of clay with dead pharaohs. Archaeologists found preserved bulbs of garlic scattered around King Tut's tomb millennia after his burial.

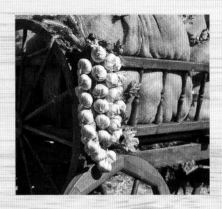

Ancient Greeks and Romans loved their garlic, too. Greek athletes and soldiers ate garlic before entering the arena or battlefield because they thought it had strength-enhancing properties. Roman soldiers ate garlic for inspiration and courage. Greek midwives hung garlic cloves in birthing rooms to repel evil spirits. Hippocrates, the ancient Greek known as the "father of medicine," prescribed garlic for a variety of ailments around 400 B.C. It was used to treat wounds, fight infection, cure leprosy, and ease digestive disorders. Other prominent Greeks used garlic to treat heart problems, as well. Garlic's reputation as a medicinal wonder continued into the Middle Ages. It was used in attempts to prevent the plague and to treat leprosy and a long list of other ailments. Later, explorers and migrating peoples introduced this easy-to-grow and easy-to-carry plant to various regions around the world. The Spanish, Portuguese, and French introduced garlic to the Americas.

For all of garlic's uses, the history of the "stinking rose" is not all rosy. In certain times and places, people despised garlic. During his reign in the 14th century, King Alphonso of Castile ordered people to stay away from him if they had eaten garlic within the past month. Its alleged aphrodisiac qualities made garlic taboo for Tibetan monks. Ancient Indians believed garlic would lure people away from spiritual endeavors, so it was banned in certain sacred places.

Garlic played its first starring role in modern medical treatment during World War I. The Russians used garlic on the front lines to treat battle wounds and fight infection, and medics used moss that was soaked in garlic as an antiseptic to pack wounds.

In the first part of the 20th century, garlic saw plenty of action off the battlefield, too. Even though penicillin was discovered in 1928, the demand for it among the general population often outstripped the supply, so many people reverted to treatments they had used with some success before, including garlic.

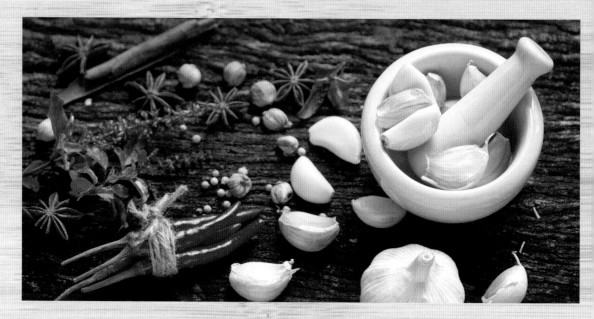

A Long Tradition in Folk Medicine

In many historic cultures, garlic was used medicinally but not in cooking. That might surprise us today, but were our ancestors able to travel into the future to visit us, they would likely think us rather dense for our culture's general lack of appreciation for the bulb's healing qualities.

Traditionally, garlic bulbs were prepared in a variety of ways for medicinal purposes. The juice of the bulb might be extracted and taken internally for one purpose, while the bulb might be ground into a paste for external treatment of other health problems. In the minds of the superstitious, simply possessing garlic was enough to bring good luck and protect against evil—especially evil in the form of mysterious and frightening entities, such as sorcerers and vampires.

Garlic in Folklore

Legends convinced people that there were certain things over which vampires had no power, and garlic was one of them. However, it is only in European (and, by extension, American) folklore that vampires are powerless in the presence of garlic. The bulb apparently is not mentioned as a defensive tool against these infamous bloodsuckers in vampire legends from other parts of the world.

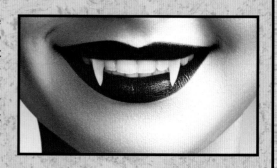

Sulfurous Substances

The pungent, ancient remedy has found its way to modern times. Herbalists have long touted garlic for a number of health problems, from preventing colds and treating intestinal problems to lowering blood cholesterol and reducing heart-disease risk. Garlic remedies abound—and scientific research has begun to support the usefulness of some of them.

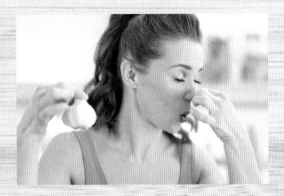

Garlic's popularity today is due in part to the efforts of scientists around the world. They have identified a number of sulfur-containing compounds in garlic that have important medicinal properties.

If you were to look at or sniff an intact garlic clove sitting on a cutting board, you'd never suspect the potent aroma and healing properties within. Whack it with a knife, however, and you open a portal. Cutting, crushing, or chewing a garlic clove activates numerous sulfurous substances. When these substances come into contact with oxygen, they form compounds that have therapeutic properties. The most researched, and possibly the most medicinally powerful, of these potent compounds are allicin and ajoene.

Garlic and Heart Health

Many studies have tried to determine whether—and how—garlic plays a role in keeping your ticker in tip-top shape. Research indicates that garlic plays a significant role in:

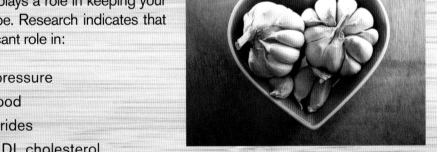

• Lowering blood pressure

• "Thinning" the blood

• Lowering triglycerides

• Lowering "bad" LDL cholesterol

• Breaking up blood clots

• Relaxing blood vessel walls and protecting them from damage

Scientists continue to research garlic's therapeutic effectiveness. Ongoing studies are gathering more data by changing the types and amounts of garlic used, the length of time participants use garlic, and the severity of participants' conditions.

Remedies for health and well-being 123

Cholesterol

Research on animals and humans in the 1980s and early 1990s seemed to indicate that garlic had much promise for lowering cholesterol. It appeared that garlic was able to lower total blood cholesterol in those who had high blood cholesterol (levels of 200 mg/dL or more). However, many of the studies included small numbers of patients and were short term, lasting just three months or less.

A number of more recent studies have tempered the initial enthusiasm about garlic's cholesterol-lowering effects. The National Center for Complementary and Alternative Medicine, a division of the National Institutes of Health (NIH), requested a thorough review of human studies that investigated garlic's ability to control cholesterol levels. The NIH released a paper in 2000 that concluded garlic did not alter HDL, but that it could significantly lower LDL cholesterol and triglycerides in the short term. Researchers determined that garlic had the greatest cholesterol-lowering effect in the first one to three months of garlic therapy. After six months, no further lipid reductions occurred.

Elevated cholesterol levels, however, contribute to heart disease over a long period of time. So based on this newer research, it would appear that although garlic may be a helpful addition to a cholesterol-lowering diet, it can't be relied on as the sole solution to high blood cholesterol levels. Still, it's obvious that more research is needed. Indeed, the NIH statement in 2000 encouraged longer-term studies, as well as consideration of the type of garlic used. For example, there is some evidence that garlic must be cut or crushed to activate its health-promoting components. But the products tested in the various studies were not consistent. Some used raw garlic, while others used dried garlic or garlic oil; sometimes the raw garlic was cut, sometimes it was minced, and sometimes it was used whole. When dried garlic was used, it often was made into a powder and formed into tablets. It's also unknown whether garlic just stops being effective after several months or whether other factors in these studies influenced the findings.

Although garlic may not be the blood-cholesterol miracle cure it was once promoted to be, and there are still plenty of questions that require answers, garlic does appear to have a healing role to play, but further studies are needed. In the meantime, however, garlic is not likely to take the place of medications prescribed by a physician to lower blood cholesterol levels. And while garlic should never take the place of prescribed medications, including it more often in a cholesterol-lowering diet is easy, inexpensive, and enhances the flavor of your meals—especially those that are low in fat and sodium.

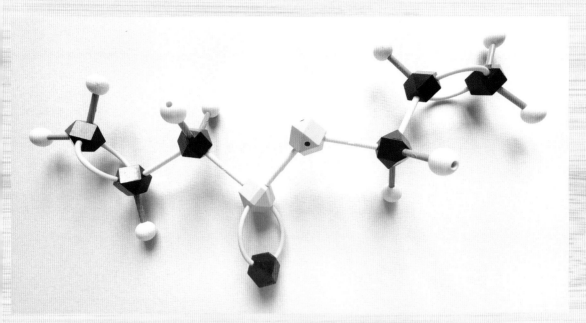

An Antioxidant Effect?

Garlic contains several powerful antioxidants—compounds that prevent oxidation, a harmful process in the body. One of them is selenium, a mineral that is a component of glutathione peroxidase, a powerful antioxidant that the body makes to defend itself. Glutathione peroxidase works with vitamin E to form a super-antioxidant defense system.

Other antioxidants in garlic include vitamin C, which helps reduce the damage that LDL cholesterol can cause, and quercetin, a phytochemical. (Phytochemicals are chemical substances found in plants that may have health benefits for people.) Garlic also has trace amounts of the mineral manganese, which is an important component of an antioxidant enzyme called superoxide dismutase.

Oxidation is related to oxygen, a vital element to every aspect of our lives, so why is oxidation so harmful? Think about when rust accumulates on your car or garden tools and eventually destroys the metal. That rust is an example of oxidation. Similarly, when your body breaks down glucose for energy, free radicals are produced. These free radicals start oxidizing—and damaging—cellular tissue. It's as if your bloodstream and blood vessels are "rusting out."

Antioxidants destroy free radicals, including those that are products of environmental factors, such as ultraviolet rays, air pollutants, cigarette smoke, rancid oils, and pesticides. The body keeps a steady supply of antioxidants ready to neutralize free radicals. Unfortunately, sometimes the number of free radicals can overwhelm the body's antioxidant stock, especially if we're not getting enough of the antioxidant nutrients.

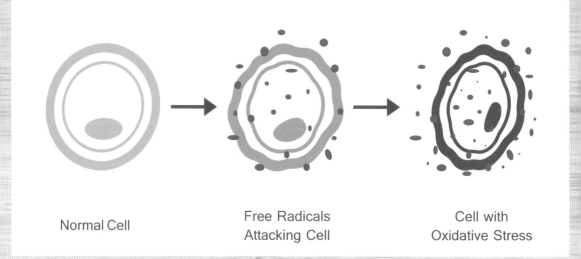

OXIDATIVE STRESS

Normal Cell   Free Radicals
Attacking Cell   Cell with
Oxidative Stress

When free radicals harm the cells that line your arteries, your body tries to mend the damage by producing a sticky spackle-like substance. However, this substance attracts cholesterol and debris that build up within the arteries, causing progressive plaque formation. The more plaque in your arteries, the more your health is in danger.

In addition, the cholesterol circulating through your arteries can be oxidized by free radicals. When LDL is oxidized, it damages the lining of the arteries, which significantly contributes to the buildup of plaque and the narrowing and hardening of the arteries.

Arteries, then, benefit greatly from the protection antioxidants provide. And garlic's ability to stop the oxidation of cholesterol may be one of the many ways it protects heart health.

Garlic also appears to help prevent calcium from binding with other substances that lodge themselves in plaque. In a UCLA Medical Center study, 19 people were given either a placebo or an aged garlic extract that contained S-allylcysteine, one of garlic's sulfur-rich compounds, for one year. The placebo group had a significantly greater increase in their calcium score (22.2 percent) than the group that received the aged garlic extract (calcium score of 7.5 percent). The results of this small pilot study suggest that aged garlic extract may inhibit the rate of coronary artery calcification. If further larger-scale studies confirm these results, garlic may prove to be a useful preventative tool for patients at high risk of future cardiovascular problems.

Blood Pressure

Research suggests that garlic can help make small improvements in blood pressure by increasing the blood flow to the capillaries, which are the tiniest blood vessels. The chemicals in garlic achieve this by causing the capillary walls to open wider and reducing the ability of blood platelets to stick together and cause blockages. Reductions are small—10 mmHg (millimeters of mercury, the unit of measurement for blood pressure) or less. This means if your blood pressure is 130 over 90 mmHg, garlic might help lower it to 120 over 80 mmHg. That's a slight improvement, but, along with some simple lifestyle adjustments, such as getting more exercise, garlic might help move your blood pressure out of the danger zone.

Infection Fighter

Garlic's potential to combat heart disease has received a lot of attention, but it should receive even more acclaim for its anti-microbial properties. Fresh, raw garlic has proven itself since ancient times as an effective killer of bacteria and viruses. Once again, we can thank allicin.

Laboratory studies confirm that raw garlic has antibacterial and antiviral properties. Not only does it knock out many common cold and flu viruses but its effectiveness also spans a broad range of both gram-positive and gram-negative bacteria (two major classifications of bacteria), fungus, intestinal parasites, and yeast. Cooking garlic, however, destroys the allicin, so you'll need to use raw garlic to prevent or fight infections.

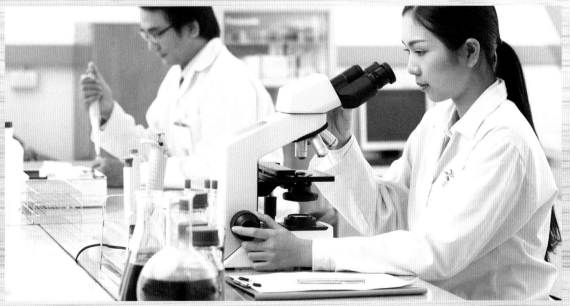

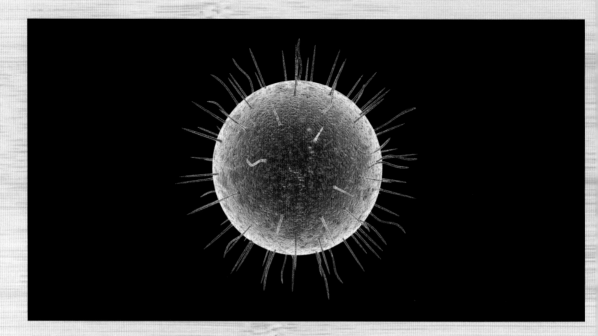

Garlic's infection-fighting capability was confirmed in a study conducted by researchers at the University of Ottawa that was published in *Phytotherapy* Research. Researchers tested 19 natural health products that contain garlic and five fresh garlic extracts for active compounds and antimicrobial activity. They tested the effectiveness of these substances against three types of common bacteria: *E. faecalis,* which causes urinary tract infections; *N. gonorrhoeae,* which causes the sexually transmitted disease gonorrhea; and *S. aureus,* which is responsible for many types of infections that are common in hospitals. The products most successful at eradicating these bacteria were the ones with the highest allicin content.

One simple but meaningful demonstration of garlic's antibacterial power can be found in a study conducted at the University of California, Irvine. Garlic juice was tested in the laboratory against a wide spectrum of potential pathogens, including several antibiotic-resistant strains of bacteria. It showed significant activity against the pathogens. Even more exciting was the fact that garlic juice still retained significant antimicrobial activity even in dilutions ranging up to 1:128 of the original juice.

Is it possible that garlic can work alongside prescription medications to reduce side effects or to help the drugs work better? Results from several studies say yes. In a Rutgers University study that used bacteria in lab dishes, garlic and two common antibiotics were pitted against certain antibiotic-resistant strains of *S. aureus* (a gram-positive bacteria) and *E. coli* (a gram-negative bacteria). Garlic was able to significantly increase the effectiveness of the two antibiotic medications in killing the bacteria.

Fighting Colds and Infections

Eating raw garlic may help combat the sickness-causing bugs that get loose inside our bodies. Garlic has been used internally as a folk remedy for years, but now the plant is being put to the test scientifically for such uses. So far, its grades are quite good as researchers pit it against a variety of bacteria.

Can a garlic clove help stop your sniffles? For eons, herbalists loaded soups and other foods with garlic and placed garlic compresses on people's chests to provide relief from colds and chest congestion. One study examined the stinking rose's ability to fight the common cold. The study involved 146 volunteers divided into two groups. One group took a garlic supplement for 12 weeks during the winter months, while the other group received a placebo. The group that received garlic had significantly fewer colds—and the colds that they did get went away faster—than the placebo group.

Garlic also may help rid the intestinal tract of Giardia lamblia, a parasite that commonly lives in stream water and causes giardiasis, an infection of the small intestine. Hikers and campers run the risk of this infection whenever they drink untreated stream or lake water. Herbalists prescribe a solution of one or more crushed garlic cloves stirred into one-third of a cup of water taken three times a day to eradicate Giardia. If you're fighting giardiasis, be sure to consult your healthcare provider, because it's a nasty infection, and ask if you can try garlic as part of your treatment.

Four Thieves' Vinegar

There are about as many versions of the four thieves' vinegar story as there are recipes for the concoction. One popular version, reported to be from the Parliament of Toulouse archives of 1628–1631, goes like this: Four thieves living in Marseilles, France, during the 17th century plagues were convicted of going to the houses of plague victims and robbing them, but the thieves themselves never became ill. How was this possible? In order to get a lesser sentence they revealed their secret—they protected themselves by consuming daily doses of a mixture that contained vinegar, garlic, and a handful of other herbs. Those in charge were so grateful that they hanged the four thieves, rather than burning them at the stake. That's gratitude for you!

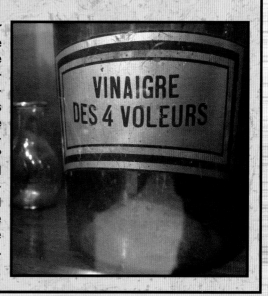

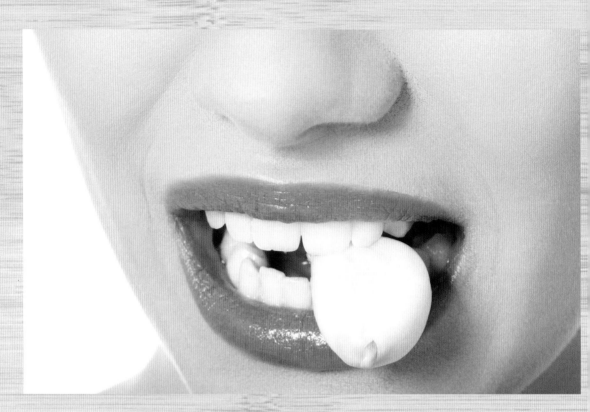

Folk Remedies Against Infection

Herbalists recommend chewing garlic and holding it in your mouth for a while before swallowing it to obtain the best dose of bacteria-fighting allicin. This may be rather difficult for children or for those who find garlic to be too spicy. As an alternative, mince a clove, let it sit for 10 to 15 minutes so the allicin can form, then stuff it into empty gelatin capsules (which you can purchase in the herb section of a natural foods store). Taking three cloves a day when you have a cold may help you feel better. If the raw garlic bothers your stomach, take the capsules with food that contains a little bit of canola oil or, better yet, olive oil.

Other folk remedies battle colds and chest congestion with a garlic poultice or plaster. To make one, put some chopped garlic in a clean cloth, thin washcloth, or paper towel. Fold it over to enclose the garlic. Pour very warm (but not hot) water over the wrapped garlic, let it sit for a few seconds, and then lightly wring it out. Place the wrapped garlic on the chest for several minutes. Reheat with very warm water and place on the back, over the lung area, for several minutes. Some herbalists also recommend placing the poultice on the soles of the feet. Caution: Be careful not to let garlic come into direct contact with the skin. Cut garlic is so powerful that prolonged exposure to the skin may result in a burn.

Anti-Inflammatory Properties

Inflammation is the body's reaction to an injury, irritation, or infection. The symptoms of inflammation include redness, swelling, and pain. Whenever the body suffers an injury, it sends many substances to the site to begin the healing process and to fight off foreign invaders, such as bacteria that can cause infections. Inflammation is so vigorous in its duties that sometimes the surrounding tissues get damaged. This can occur at the site of a wound, inside blood vessels that have succumbed to an injury by oxidized LDL cholesterol, or in airways that are exposed to something that irritates them.

Certain complexes in garlic appear to help minimize the body's inflammatory response. By decreasing inflammation, garlic may lend a hand by doing the following:

• Protecting the inside of your arteries
• Reducing the severity of asthma
• Protecting against inflammation in the joints, such as in rheumatoid arthritis and osteoarthritis
• Reducing inflammation in nasal passages and airways, such as that associated with colds

Anti-Cancer Properties

Some scientists think garlic may be able to help prevent one of the most dreaded maladies—cancer. The Mayo Clinic has reported that some studies using cancer cells in the laboratory, as well as some studies with animals and people, have suggested that eating garlic, especially unprocessed garlic, might reduce the risk of stomach and colon cancers.

The National Institutes of Health's National Cancer Institute drew similar conclusions after reviewing 37 studies involving garlic and sulfur-containing compounds. Twenty-eight of those studies indicated garlic possessed at least some anticancer activity, especially toward prostate and stomach cancer. Because the studies in question were merely observational (they compared people who reported eating a lot of garlic to those who did not), more studies are needed.

Still, the research the National Cancer Institute reviewed found that it may not take much garlic to reap these anticancer benefits. Eating as few as two servings of garlic a week might be enough to help protect against colon cancer. Controlled clinical trials will help determine the true extent of garlic's cancer-fighting powers.

What gives garlic this wonderful gift? Several factors, including antioxidants and those same sulfur-containing agents we've discussed before, including allicin. (Antioxidants help protect cells from damage; continual cell damage can eventually lead to cancer.) Allicin appears to protect colon cells from the toxic effects of cancer-causing agents. For instance, when meat is cooked with garlic, the herb reduces the production of cancer-causing compounds that would otherwise form when meat is grilled at high temperatures.

Garlic's potential ability to decrease *H. pylori* bacteria in the stomach may help prevent gastritis (inflammation of the stomach lining) from eventually evolving into cancer. (*H. pylori* is most famous for its link to stomach ulcers, but it can also cause chronic gastritis.) Numerous studies around the world indicate that garlic's sulfur-containing compounds have the potential to help prevent stomach cancer.

Most studies do not show a reduction in breast cancer risk related to garlic intake. The data about whether garlic helps prevent development of prostate cancer is less definitive. And in a preliminary study that looked at consumption of fruits and vegetables, garlic appeared to be the only variable that might slightly decrease the risk of ovarian cancer; clearly, however, more studies are needed.

Cancer-Fighting Compounds

Crushing, chopping, or chewing garlic releases a host of cancer-fighting compounds, including some with names you might recognize and some that may not be familiar. They include:

- allicin
- alliin
- alline
- ajoene, a disulfide
- diallyl disulfide (DADS)
- diallyl sulfide (DAS)
- diallyl trisulfide (DAT)
- quercetin (a phytochemical that is a potent antioxidant)
- S-allylcysteine (SAC)
- selenium (a mineral that is part of an antioxidant complex made by the body)
- vitamin C (has proven antioxidant activity)

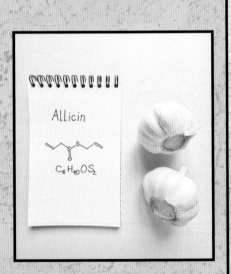

Allicin

$C_6H_{10}OS_2$

Supplements

Fresh, naturally grown raw garlic is best, but if you can't get enough of it into your diet, here is the scoop on supplements. Not all garlic supplements consistently have the amount of allicin claimed on the label when they undergo testing. There are many possible variables, including differences in the garlic itself, growing conditions, amounts and types of fertilizer, type of garlic, the processing methods used, and quality control during manufacturing.

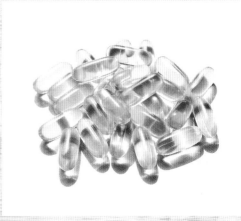

This remains a problem with assessing research on garlic—do the commercial garlic preparations contain what they say they do? Which compounds do they really have and how much is there in the supplement you're taking?

Supplements are typically made by slicing garlic and drying it at low temperatures to prevent the destruction of alliinase, the enzyme that turns alliin into the disease-fighter allicin. It is then pulverized into a powder and formed into tablets. In order to meet the standards set by the U.S. Pharmacopeia (the group that develops the quality standards for prescription and over-the-counter drugs and dietary supplements sold in the United States), the powder must contain at least 0.3 percent alliin.

Because manufacturers process and label their supplements differently, shopping for garlic supplements can be confusing. Some tablets do not contain any allicin, but rather alliin, which is converted to allicin. Other tablets contain both alliin and allicin. And some supplement labels may have an "allicin potential" or "allicin yield" statement. This refers to the amount of allicin that could be formed when alliin is converted, not how much allicin is actually formed.

In addition, because the enzyme alliinase is destroyed by the strong acidic conditions in the stomach, most supplements are "enteric coated" to keep them from dissolving until they reach the small intestine. Most tablets tested, though, produce only a little allicin under these tough conditions, and the tablets often take too long to dissolve. The better measurement is "allicin release." This discloses how much allicin the supplement actually produces under conditions similar to those found in the digestive tract. However, only a few manufacturers list this measurement on their labels.

With all this in mind, you should start by looking for the "standardization" statement on a label when choosing a garlic supplement—but even this isn't a foolproof guarantee. When a product is "standardized" it is supposed to have a certain amount of a specific ingredient. For instance, a product that says, "standardized to contain 1.3 percent alliin" means that every pill in every bottle should contain at least 1.3 percent alliin. Unfortunately, this is not always the case, but a product that carries the USP (U.S. Pharmacopeia) seal follows set methods to help ensure standardization.

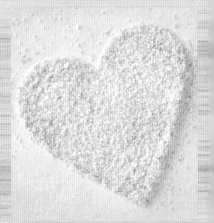

Allicin is not the only active compound in garlic, but the other compounds are typically not standardized. Thus, you often don't know everything you're getting when purchasing a supplement.

Which kind of supplement is best? Dried garlic powder is considered to have effects similar to those of fresh, crushed garlic. Other types of supplements, such as oils from crushed garlic, aged garlic extract in alcohol, and steam-distilled oils seem to contain less allicin and perhaps less of other active compounds than the dried powder.

When shopping for a garlic supplement, look for one that indicates it is standardized to contain at least 1.3 percent allicin. In the United States, pharmacy-grade garlic contains 0.3 percent (powdered form) to 0.5 percent (fresh, dried form) allicin. Avoid enteric-coated or time-release tablets because these may not dissolve soon enough in your digestive tract to make use of the allicin.

Clove vs. Supplement

Rather than fussing over garlic supplements that may or may not contain what they claim, just enjoy the heady aroma and flavor of fresh garlic in the foods you eat. You'll always know you're getting the best—and the most potent—allicin you can when you add garlic to foods. Consider this:

• A typical garlic clove weighs about 3 grams.

• The amount of alliin in an average clove ranges from 24 milligrams to 56 milligrams.

• A standard clove will produce about 2.5 milligrams to 4.5 milligrams of allicin per gram of fresh weight when crushed. This means you'll get 7.5 milligrams to 13.5 milligrams of allicin from one typical clove that weighs 3 grams.

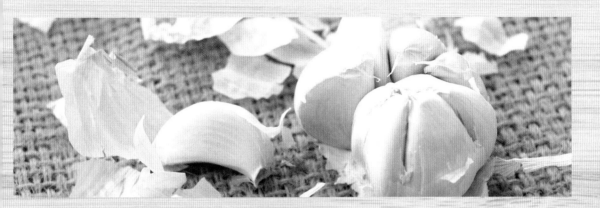

Peeling and Use

To easily peel garlic, slice off each end of a clove. Then, turn your broad chef's knife sideways so the flat side is parallel to your cutting board and the sharp edge is facing away from you. Place your knife this way on top of the clove and give the blade a quick pop with the heel of your hand to lightly crush the garlic clove (you don't want to mash it). The papery skins then rub off easily.

If you're going to peel many garlic cloves at once, drop them into boiling water for 10 to 20 seconds. Then plunge them into cold water. The skins will slide right off between your thumb and forefinger.

To separate the individual cloves from the bulb, place the bulb on a flat surface. Use the heel of your hand to apply firm but gentle pressure at an angle. The parchment layers will separate, allowing you to carefully remove as many cloves as you need. Then, tenderly remove the thin covering on each individual clove. Most people reach for the plumpest cloves, but the smaller cloves have a more intense flavor.

Whether you rule garlic with a gentle or firm hand determines the amount and type of flavor you get. Here are some taste tips:

• Gently peel and use cloves whole to impart just a hint of garlic flavor.

• Slice cloves lengthwise for mild flavor or for those long-cooking dishes.

• Mince cloves for medium flavor or for your quick-cooking dishes.

• Firmly push cloves through a garlic press for the strongest flavor. If you don't have a garlic press, put your knife to work and finely chop the garlic. Remember, the smaller the pieces, the more pungent the flavor. Sprinkle the chopped garlic with a bit of salt, because salt pulls out liquid from the chopped garlic. Then firmly rub the salted chopped garlic with the side of your knife blade, further crushing it.

Remedies for health and well-being 135

Getting the Most from Garlic

Because one of garlic's most beneficial ingredients, allicin, is partially destroyed by cooking, you'll get the greatest health boost if you use it raw or only lightly cooked when you can. However, cooking garlic forms other healthful sulfur compounds, so you still receive benefits when you cook it. Plan ahead so you can cut, crush, or chop your garlic and let it sit for 15 minutes or more before using it to activate the enzymes that turn alliin into allicin.

Ideas for Use

Garlic adds the spice of life to foods in countries all around the world. Along with ginger and onions, garlic flavors many of the foods of Southeast Asia. Teamed with tahini, it makes Middle-Eastern foods dining delights. Combined with chili peppers, garlic adds spark to Latin cuisine. You can make a simple bruschetta that's a great appetizer with olive oil, capers, tomato, and cheese. Roast garlic with cheese makes a fantastic dip. Bake 2 heads of garlic at 400 degrees Fahrenheit for about 45 minutes, then mash and add goat cheese, blue cheese, or both. Serve with vegetables. Roasted garlic cloves also add great flavor to chicken.

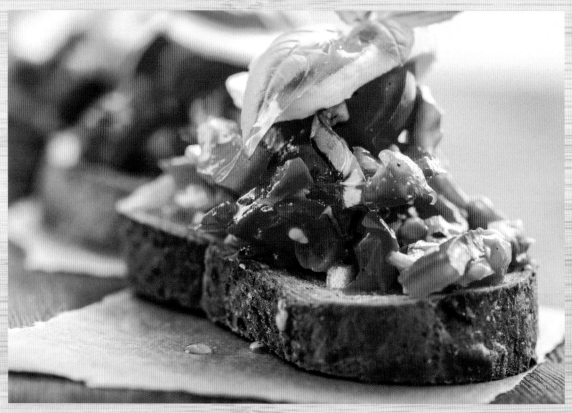

Cautions

Garlic is safe for most adults. Other than that special aroma garlic lends to your breath and perspiration, the herb has few side effects. However, you should know about a few cautions:

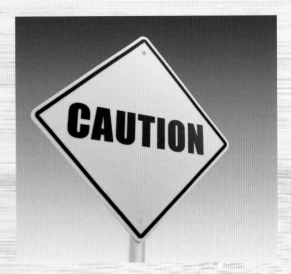

• If you are allergic to plants in the Liliaceae (lily) family, including onions, leeks, chives, and such flowers as hyacinth and tulip, avoid garlic. People who are allergic to garlic may have reactions whether it's taken by mouth, inhaled, or applied to the skin.

• People anticipating surgery or dental procedures, pregnant women, and those with bleeding disorders should avoid taking large amounts of garlic on a regular basis due to its ability to "thin" the blood, which could cause excessive bleeding. Taking blood thinners such as warfarin (brand name Coumadin) or aspirin and other non-steroidal anti-inflammatory drugs (such as ibuprofen or naproxen) along with garlic is not recommended unless you first discuss it with your health-care provider so dosing adjustments can be made. To be safe, if you have any questions about your use of garlic, talk with your health-care provider.

• Garlic interferes with medications other than anticoagulants. Garlic may interact with and affect the action of birth control pills, cyclosporine (often prescribed for rheumatoid arthritis), and some other medications. It also interferes with certain HIV/AIDS antiviral medications, reducing their effectiveness. Talk with your health-care provider and/or pharmacist if you take prescription medications and regularly eat large amounts of garlic or take any type of garlic supplement.

• Nursing women may find that garlic gives their milk an "off" flavor that the baby may reject, resulting in shorter nursing times.

• Consuming large amounts of garlic can irritate the stomach lining and possibly cause heartburn, abdominal pain, flatulence, diarrhea, or constipation. Go easy with garlic if you have a sensitive stomach.

• If applied directly to the skin, garlic can cause burns. Be especially careful using raw garlic on children's skin.

Sesame Noodle Bowl

- 1 package (16 ounces) uncooked spaghetti
- 6 tablespoons soy sauce
- 5 tablespoons dark sesame oil
- 3 tablespoons sugar
- 3 tablespoons rice vinegar
- 4 tablespoons vegetable oil, divided
- 3 cloves garlic, minced
- 1 teaspoon grated fresh ginger or ginger paste
- ½ teaspoon sriracha sauce
- 2 green onions, sliced
- 1 red bell pepper, cut into thin strips
- 1 cucumber
- 1 carrot
- 1 package (14 to 16 ounces) firm tofu, drained and patted dry

***Sesame seeds (optional)

1. Cook spaghetti according to package directions until al dente in large saucepan of boiling salted water. Drain, reserving 1 tablespoon pasta cooking water.

2. Whisk soy sauce, sesame oil, sugar, vinegar, 2 tablespoons vegetable oil, garlic, ginger and sriracha in large bowl. Stir in noodles, reserved pasta cooking water and green onions. Let stand at least 30 minutes until noodles have cooled to room temperature and most of sauce is absorbed, stirring occasionally.

3. Meanwhile, cut bell pepper into thin strips. Peel cucumber and carrot and shred with julienne peeler into long strands, or cut into thin strips.

4. Cut tofu into thin triangles or 1-inch cubes. Heat remaining 2 tablespoons oil in large nonstick skillet over high heat. Add tofu; cook 5 minutes or until browned on all sides, turning occasionally.

5. Place noodles in bowls. Top with tofu, bell pepper, cucumber and carrot. Sprinkle with sesame seeds, if desired.

Note: Sesame noodles are great served warm or cold. To serve them cold, cover and refrigerate a few hours or overnight after step 2 before preparing the vegetables and tofu. For a side dish or potluck dish, skip the tofu and stir the vegetables into the noodles after they are cool. Refrigerate until ready to serve.

Makes 6 servings

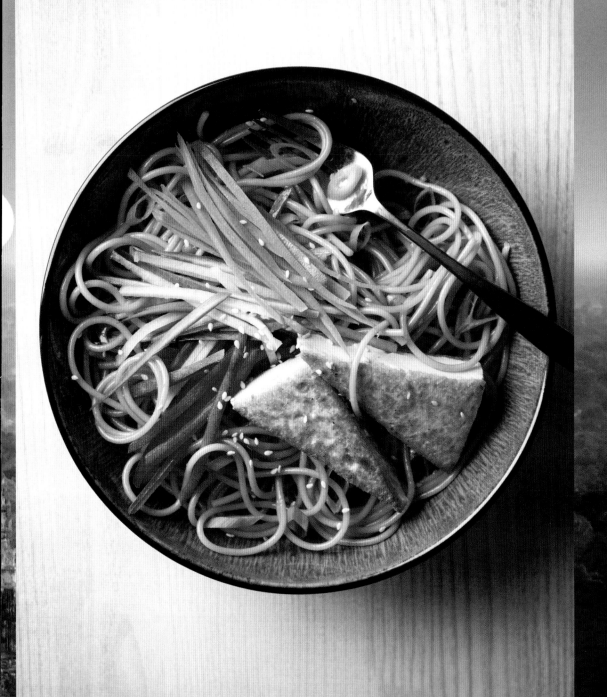

Ginger

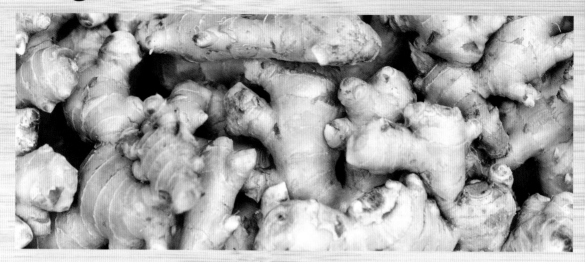

Most every child knows the taste of ginger. It's the prime ingredient in ginger ale, ginger-bread, and gingersnaps. Used fresh, or dried and powdered for a culinary spice, it is a major ingredient in curries and other Eastern cuisines. The Chinese scholar Confucius ate fresh ginger with every meal. Since it was one of the earliest herbs transported in the spice trade, it is now difficult to determine if ginger originated in India or China. But the popular kitchen spice enjoys a rich history as a medicinal aid as well.

Health Benefits

Ginger is a potent anti-nausea medication, useful for treating morning sickness, motion sickness, and nausea accompanying gastroenteritis (stomach "flu"). As a stomach calming aid, ginger reduces gas, bloating, and indigestion and aids in the body's absorption of nutrients and other herbs. Ginger is also a valuable deterrent to several types of intestinal worms. And the herb may work as a therapy and preventive treatment for some migraine headaches and rheumatoid arthritis.

Ginger promotes perspiration if ingested in large amounts. Use internally or topically. The herb stimulates circulation, so if you are cold, you can use warm ginger tea to help raise your body heat. Ginger may occasionally promote menstrual flow. It also prevents platelets from clumping and thins the blood, which reduces the risk of atherosclerosis and blood clots. Grated ginger poultices or compresses ease lung congestion when placed on the chest and alleviate gas, nausea, and menstrual cramps when laid on the abdomen.

Small studies have used ginger extracts to treat pain or inflammation caused by arthritis.

Home Remedies

As an expectorant for bronchitis: Steep ½ teaspoon ginger, a pinch of ground cloves, and a pinch of cinnamon in 1 cup boiling water.

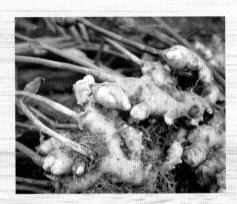

Ginger can stimulate a poor appetite. Try some ginger tea or gingersnaps, or chop up some fresh ginger and mix it with a little lime juice and a pinch of rock salt, then chew. It will not only increase appetite but thirst, too.

Ginger does contain anti-inflammatory compounds, including some with mild aspirinlike effects. When your back aches, cut a 1- to 2-inch fresh ginger root into slices and place in 1 quart boiling water. Simmer, covered, for 30 minutes on low heat. Cool for 30 minutes. Strain, sweeten with honey (to taste), and drink.

Ginger tea can help relieve the need to belch. Pour 1 cup boiling water over 1 teaspoon freshly grated gingerroot. Steep for 5 minutes, then drink. Or mix 1 teaspoon fresh ginger pulp with 1 teaspoon lime juice, and take after eating.

Ginger, which has antiviral properties, shares the limelight with licorice in this cough remedy. To make ginger-licorice (anise) tea, combine 2 teaspoons freshly chopped gingerroot, 2 teaspoons aniseed, and if available, 1 teaspoon dried licorice root in 2 cups boiling water. Cover and steep for ten minutes. Strain and sweeten with 1 or 2 teaspoons honey. Drink ½ cup every one to two hours, but no more than 3 cups a day.

One hour before flying, drink a cup of ginger tea to soothe your nerves and provide last-minute hydration.

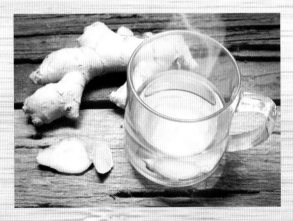

This can help break a high fever. Grate 2 tablespoons fresh ginger and add to 2 cups boiling water. Steep 30 minutes. Add a little honey to sweeten, and drink a cup of the warm beverage every two to three hours.

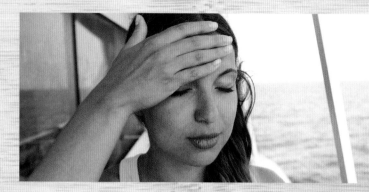

Ginger has long been used to treat nausea and seasickness. And, since having a hangover is much like being seasick, this easy remedy works wonders. If you're really green, the best bet is to drink ginger ale (no preparation required). If you can remain vertical for ten minutes, brew some ginger tea. Cut 10 to 12 slices of fresh ginger root and combine with 4 cups water. Boil for ten minutes. Strain and add the juice of 1 orange, the juice of ½ lemon, and ½ cup honey. Drink to your relief.

A tea from this root can soothe heartburn. Add 1½ teaspoons ginger root to 1 cup water; simmer for ten minutes. Drink as needed.

When you have laryngitis, fragrant, fresh ginger can help soothe inflamed mucous membranes of the larynx. Try sucking on candied ginger if available or drink a cup of ginger tea. To prepare the tea, cut a fresh 1- to 2-inch gingerroot into thin slices and place in 1 quart boiling water. Cover the pot and simmer on the lowest heat for 30 minutes. Let cool for 30 more minutes, strain, and drink ½ to 1 cup three to five times a day. Sweeten with honey if needed.

Ginger has long been known as an herbal remedy for queasiness, but modern science has proved this spice has merit, especially for motion sickness. One study discovered that ginger was actually better than over-the-counter motion sickness drugs. Make a ginger tea to take along with you when you're traveling. You could also try candied ginger: a one-inch piece should do the trick. And there's also enough ginger in gingersnaps and ginger ale to ease milder bouts of nausea.

Warning! For queasiness caued by morning sickness, consult your doctor. Ginger has been used in folk medicine as a remedy for morning sickness, but some experts frown upon using ginger during pregnancy. Should you have any doubts, consult your doctor.

For a sore throat, mix 2 parts cinnamon, 2 parts ginger, and 3 parts licorice powder. Steep 1 teaspoon of this mixture in 1 cup boiling water for ten minutes, then drink as a sore throat cure three times a day.

Ideas for Use

Ginger is a staple of many cuisines, including those of southeast Asia, India, Japan, the Caribbean, and North Africa. Add the spicy chopped root to beverages, fruits, meats, fish, preserves, pickles, and a variety of vegetables. Use ground ginger in breads, cookies, and other desserts.

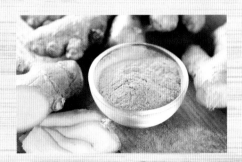

Essential Oil

Use a ginger compress wrapped around the neck or placed on the chest to ease sore throat or lung congestion. The smell of it alone will often open congested sinuses. If you experience nausea or motion sickness, inhale a drop placed on a hankie. To relieve indigestion or menstrual cramps, rub a massage oil containing ginger into the skin on your abdomen or place a poultice made from the grated root on it. In a warming liniment, ginger essential oil treats poor circulation and sore or cramped muscles, since it decreases the substances in the body that make muscles cramp.

Migraine Headache Hand Soak

- 5 drops lavender oil
- 5 drops ginger oil
- 1 quart hot water, about 110°

Add essential oils to the hot water, and soak hands for at least 3 minutes. This therapy can be done repeatedly.

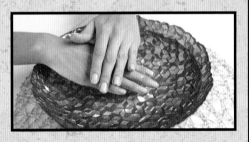

Cautions

Although ginger is prescribed for nausea, some people develop this symptom after ingesting very large amounts. People on blood thinners should consult their doctor before taking ginger medicinally. Ginger essential oil is a known dermal irritant. Be careful while handling it and do not use again if you experience a skin reaction. Even if the reaction is mild, sensitization and a more severe reaction can occur with repeated use.

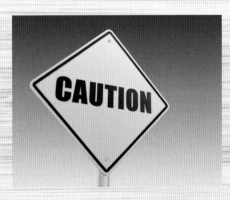

Cedar Plank Salmon with Grilled Citrus Mango

- 4 salmon fillets (6 ounces each), skin intact
- 2 teaspoons sugar, divided
- 1 teaspoon chili powder
- ½ teaspoon black pepper
- ¼ teaspoon salt
- ¼ teaspoon ground allspice
- 2 tablespoons orange juice
- 1 tablespoon lemon juice
- 1 tablespoon lime juice
- 2 teaspoons minced fresh ginger
- ¼ cup chopped fresh mint
- ⅛ teaspoon red pepper flakes
- 2 medium mangoes, peeled and cut into 1-inch pieces
- 1 cedar plank (about 15X7 inches, ½ inch thick), soaked*

1. Prepare grill for direct cooking over medium-high heat.

2. Rinse and pat dry salmon fillets. Combine 1 teaspoon sugar, chili powder, black pepper, salt and allspice in small bowl. Rub evenly over flesh side of fillets. Set aside.

3. Combine remaining 1 teaspoon sugar, orange, lemon and lime juices, ginger, mint and red pepper flakes in medium bowl; mix well.

4. Thread mango pieces onto skewers or spread out in grill basket.

5. If using charcoal grill, wait until coals are covered with gray ash to start grilling salmon. If using gas grill, turn heat down to medium. Keep clean spray bottle filled with water nearby in case plank begins to burn. If it flares up, spray lightly with water.

6. Lightly brush grid with oil and place soaked plank on top. Cover, heat until plank smokes and crackles. Place salmon, skin side down, on plank and arrange mango skewers alongside plank. Cover. Grill 6 to 8 minutes, turning skewers frequently, until mango pieces are slightly charred. Remove mango from the grill; set aside. Cover; grill salmon 9 to 12 minutes or until the flesh begins to flake when tested with fork.

7. Remove plank from grill and transfer salmon to serving platter. Slide mango pieces off skewers and add to mint mixture, tossing gently to coat. Serve immediately alongside salmon.

Tip: Cedar planks can be purchased at gourmet kitchen stores or hardware stores. Be sure to buy untreated wood at least ½ inch thick. Use each plank for grilling food only once. Used planks may be broken up into wood chips and used to smoke foods.

Makes 4 servings

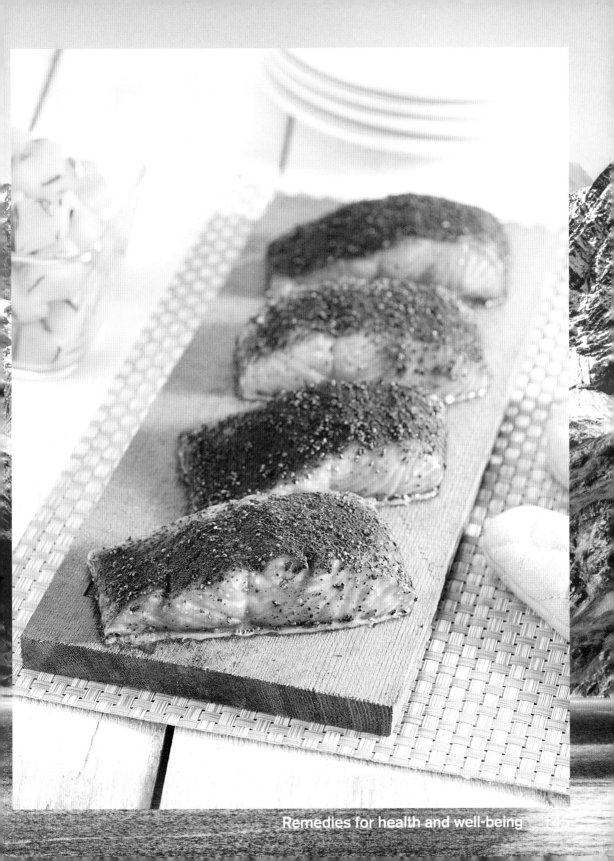

Ginseng

The Chinese have used a close relative of American ginseng (*Panax quinquefolius*) since prehistoric times. In the United States, colonists grew rich collecting American ginseng and exporting it to China, where the herb enjoys a strong reputation as an aphrodisiac and prolonger of life. Ginseng is an adaptogen, capable of protecting the body from physical and mental stress and helping bodily functions return to normal.

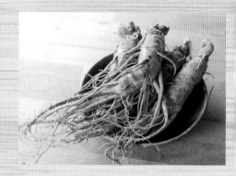

What It Looks Like

American ginseng produces a single stem, a whorl of leaves, and several green-white flowers from June through August. Leaves are toothed; the berries, bright red. American ginseng is indigenous to Manitoba and Quebec and ranges south to Georgia and west through Alabama to Oklahoma. It may be found in hardwood forests on north or northwestern slopes, although years of high demand have made it scarce in the wild.

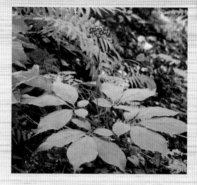

Ginseng needs to be pampered but can be grown in home gardens. The herb demands shade and humusy, rich, well-drained loam. Commercially, ginseng is grown in shelters that mimic forests. The plant must be mulched in winter and takes from five to seven years to produce usable roots, which often fall prey to rotting diseases or gophers. Ginseng seeds require a cold period of at least four months to germinate. The most common way to grow it is to buy seedlings two to three years old. Do not uproot this endangered plant if you're lucky enough to find it growing wild. Purchase products made from cultivated ginseng, or grow your ginseng. Dry the roots or preserve them in alcohol or honey.

Health Benefits

Clinical studies indicate that ginseng may slow the effects of aging, protect cells from free radical damage, prevent heart disease, and help treat anemia, atherosclerosis, depression, diabetes, edema (excess fluid buildup), ulcers, and hypertension. Its complex saponins, ginsenosides, are responsible for most of its actions. Purportedly, they stimulate bone marrow production and immune system functions, inhibit tumor growth, and detoxify the liver. Ginseng has many dual roles, for example, raising or lowering blood pressure or blood sugar, according to the body's needs.

Ginseng gently stimulates and strengthens the central nervous system, making it useful for treating fatigue and weakness caused by disease and injury. It reduces mental confusion and headaches.

Folk Remedies

For anxiety, simmer the root on low heat in enough water to cover the root twice. When half the water is evaporated, remove from heat to cool. Strain and drink twice a day. You can also buy ginseng extracts that readily dissolve in hot water.

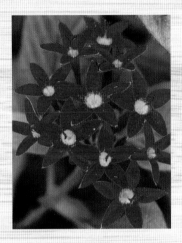

Drinking a ginseng wine may help sleepless nights, especially if they're related to stress or a fever-producing illness. Chop 3½ ounces ginseng (use only American ginseng) and place in 1 quart liquor, such as vodka. Let it stand for five to six weeks in a cool, dark place. Turn the container frequently. Take 1 ounce before bed.

Ginseng is an age-old energy booster. This root has a sweet licorice taste and has been used for thousands of years to treat weakness and exhaustion. Be cautious: Don't take ginseng unless you are really fatigued. It can be too stimulating if you're feeling fine. In America you're probably wise to buy Asian ginseng. Another variety, Siberian ginseng, may not be as potent as the Asian variety. You can buy ginseng powder at a reputable herb shop. Take 2 grams of ginseng powder a day for a six-week stint. Then take at least a two-week break before using the energizing herb again.

Dosages

Herbalists recommend taking about 1 gram of dried root per day. This amount is equivalent to about 4 capsules or 1 to 2 teaspoons tincture (4 to 8 droppers full). Or chew on the whole root. It is also available in a thick concentrated extract to make instant tea and as a sweetened liquid extract. Some herbalists recommend that you take ginseng for several weeks, then stop using it for a week or two for optimum effects.

Cautions

Ginseng is generally considered safe. Side effects of taking quantities of ginseng or mixing it with large amounts of caffeine may include some of the symptoms for which it is prescribed, including insomnia, nervousness, and irritability. Consult a physician or qualified herbalist before using ginseng if you have high blood pressure or are pregnant. Use of ginseng aggravates some cases of hypertension and improves other cases.

Horseradish

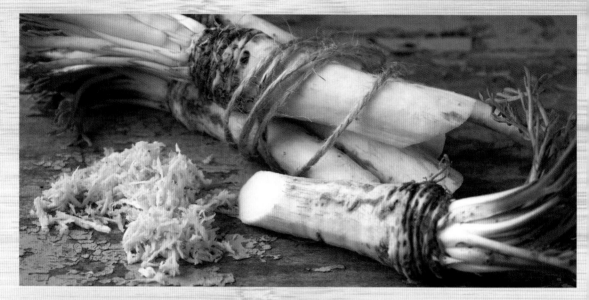

Have you ever bitten into a roast beef sandwich and thought your nose was on fire? The sandwich probably contained horseradish. Even a tiny taste of this potent condiment seems to go straight to your nose. Whether it's on a roast beef sandwich or in an herbal preparation, horseradish clears sinuses, increases circulation, and promotes expulsion of mucus from upper respiratory passages.

The Plant

Horseradish, a cousin of mustard, produces a long tapering root. Its flowers are small and white and appear in midsummer; its leaves are abundant. Native to southeastern Europe and western Asia, the herb is cultivated widely in North America and naturalized in some areas. It's easy to care for, too, if you'd ever like to grow your own. And you don't need to worry that your garden will smell—the pungent odor develops when the flesh of the root is crushed. The compound allyl isothiocyanate helps protect the plant from herbivores; it's also what gives horseradish its flavor. Horseradish prefers average, moist, heavy soil and full sun. Once established, it is difficult to eradicate. Some gardeners believe that planting horseradish near potatoes makes them more disease resistant.

To preserve horseradish, harvest the roots in late fall. Store whole in dry sand in a cool, dark place. Horseradish roots will stay fresh for months. The best way to preserve horseradish is to put it in vinegar or lemon juice right after grating it; the mustard oil produced upon grating is quickly lost otherwise. Use grated horseradish within three months. Reconstitute dried horseradish at least 30 minutes before serving.

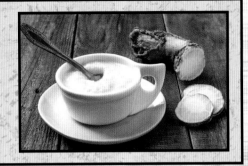

Prepared Horseradish

Peel and grate horseradish root until you have about one cup. Mix it with ¾ cup vinegar and ¼ teaspoon salt in a blender. The flavor will often strengthen over the first few days.

Health Benefits

Horseradish has been used as a medicine for centuries. Its chief constituent decomposes upon exposure to air to turn into mustard oil, which gives both horseradish and mustard their heat and flavor. The root contains an antibiotic substance and vitamin C, which are effective in clearing up sinus, bronchial, and urinary infections. Horseradish can make an effective heat-producing poultice that alleviates the pain of arthritis and neuralgia. It also stimulates digestion and has long been eaten with fatty foods to help digest them.

Horseradish has also been used to treat urinary tract infections, kidney stones, gallbladder disorders, and sciatic nerve pain. There is some scientific evidence to back up the idea that bronchitis, sinus, and urinary tract infections can be helped by horseradish. Evidence is scarcer for other uses.

Fresh root is superior as both medicine and food, but dried horseradish powder will do in a pinch.

Prepared horseradish has little fat, so it's recommended as a tasty topping for those trying to lose weight or for people with diabetes who are trying to avoid creamy sauces.

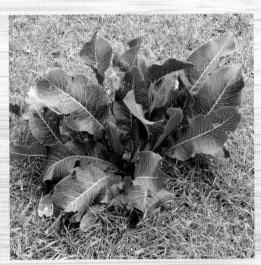

Horseradish is a cruciferous vegetable, like broccoli and cauliflower. Some recent research has noted that horseradish contain glucosinolates, as do many cruciferous vegetables, which may have protective effects against cancer. One 2016 study noted that horseradish contains 10 times the level of glucosinolates than broccoli.

Home Remedies

Stir horseradish in a sip of warm water with a little honey and take for hoarseness or head congestion, or take ½ teaspoon tincture (2 droppers full) in warm water. Repeat every hour until the problem clears.

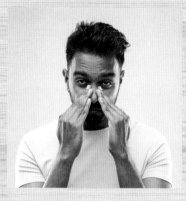

Try this Russian sore throat cure. Combine 1 tablespoon pure horseradish or horseradish root with 1 teaspoon honey and 1 teaspoon ground cloves. Mix in a glass of warm water and drink slowly.

If you're a hay fever sufferer and sushi lover combined, this remedy will please. Wasabi, that pale-green, fiery condiment served alongside California rolls, is a member of the horseradish family. Anyone who has taken too big a dollop of wasabi or plain old horseradish knows how it makes sinuses and tear ducts spring into action. That's because allyl isothiocyanate promotes phlegm flow and has antiasthmatic properties. The tastiest way to get in those allyl isothiocyanates is by slathering horseradish on your sandwich or plopping wasabi onto your favorite sushi. The last, harder-to-swallow option is to purchase grated horseradish and take ¼ teaspoon during an allergy attack.

Wonderful Wasabi

Japanese wasabi grows primarily in Japan and is often called Japanese horseradish. In wasabi preparations outside Japan, western horseradish is often used. However, you might be able to find Japanese horseradish at your local Asian grocery store. Wash the root, remove its leaves and any marks, and grate the root to make wasabi. You can also buy wasabi powder and reconstitute it with water to make paste.

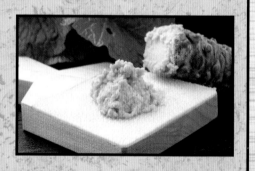

Horseradish can also be used to open up the sinus in the case of bronchitis. Be careful not to use horseradish if you're having stomach problems, though, because it's too potent. Eat it straight, on a salad, or atop meat. Fresh horseradish is the best choice, but commercial products will work, too. Make sure it's straight horseradish, though. Sandwich spreads with horseradish won't work. One study showed that a combination of horseradish root and nasturtium treated the symptoms of bronchitis as well as antibiotics.

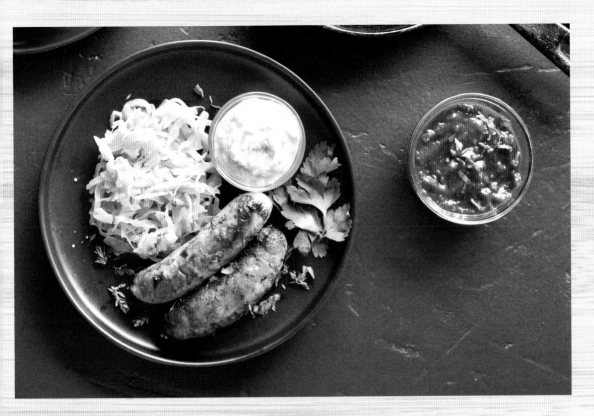

Ideas for Use

As a condiment, horseradish is widely used. Its sharp mustardy taste enhances mayonnaise, fish, beef, sausage, eggs, potatoes, and beets. Horseradish is used extensively in Eastern European cuisine and is a featured ingredient in Dresden sauce. Tender new leaves may be chopped fine and tossed in salads.

Grate the fresh root in a food processor or blender. Add vinegar and honey or sugar to taste. Spread ¼ teaspoon or less of prepared horseradish on a cracker and eat it.

Mix horseradish with its relative mustard for an extra kick. Tewkesbury mustard, an English condiment mentioned as far back as Shakespeare, is a combination of both.

Cautions

Large doses of horseradish may cause an upset stomach, vomiting, or headache. Topical use may cause inflammation. Horseradish's volatile fumes may irritate the lungs if you inhale large quantities on a continuous basis.

Beefy Stuffed Mushrooms

- 1 pound 90% lean ground beef
- 2 teaspoons prepared horseradish
- 1 teaspoon chopped fresh chives
- 1 clove garlic, minced
- ¼ teaspoon black pepper
- 18 large mushrooms
- ⅔ cup dry white wine

1. Preheat oven to 350°F. Combine beef, horseradish, chives, garlic and pepper in medium bowl; mix well.

2. Remove stems from mushrooms; fill caps with beef mixture.

3. Place stuffed mushrooms in shallow baking dish; pour wine over mushrooms. Bake 20 minutes or until meat is browned and cooked through.

Makes 1½ dozen mushrooms

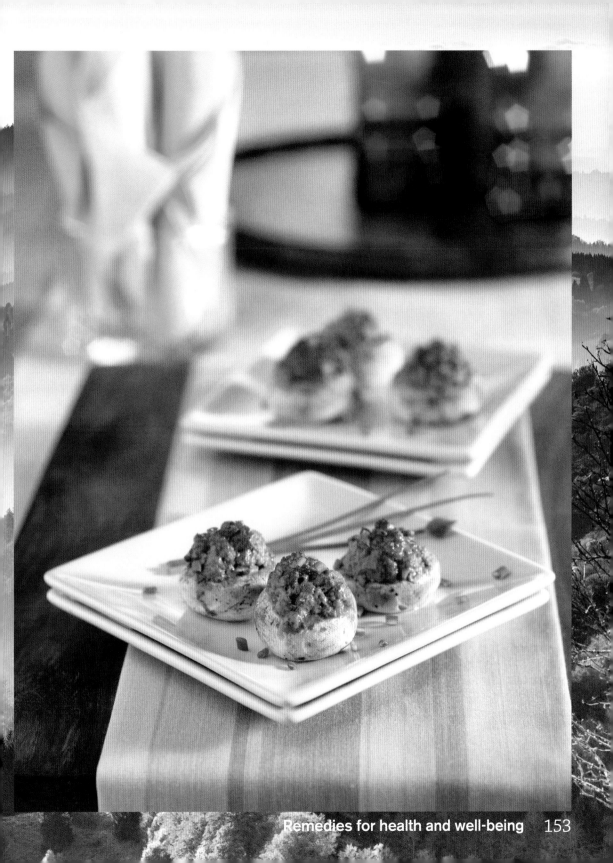

Mustard

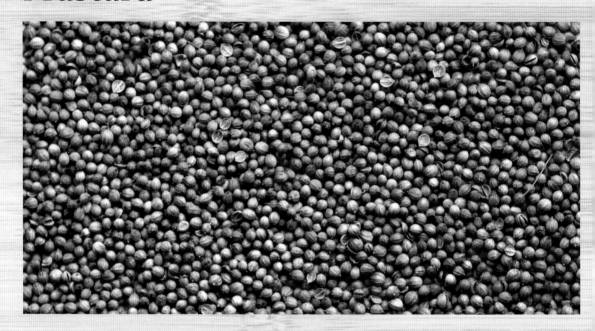

Can something you're used to eating on hot dogs and hamburgers help you out? Maybe! Mustard the condiment takes its name from its chief ingredient, the seeds of the mustard plant. It's been used as a condiment since the days of the Romans, who mixed mustard seeds with grape juice. From Rome the condiment spread to France, and the city of Dijon in particular became a famous center of mustard making in the Middle Ages. The specific recipe we recognize now as Dijon mustard was popularized in the 1800s; it combines mustard seeds with white wine or wine vinegar, water, and salt. The yellow mustard popular in America gets its color from—drum roll please—turmeric.

The Mustard Plant

You'll recognize species of the large mustard family by their strong smell and four-petaled flowers. Mustard flowers are small and yellow, and the petals resemble a Maltese cross. Lower leaves are pinnately lobed or coarsely toothed; upper leaves are not as lobed. The plant flowers in early summer. Mustards grow just about everywhere. These are hardy plants. White mustard grows wild throughout the world and has many cousins, including cabbage, broccoli, and turnips.

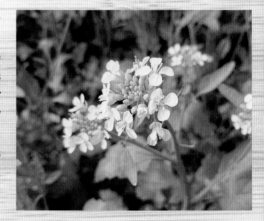

Cultivation

Did you know you could grow your own plants and make your own mustard? Plant mustard seeds 1/8 inch deep in a sunny spot, where the soil is average to poor and well drained. Yellow mustard tolerates heavy soil conditions better than black mustard. Thin seedlings to about 9 inches apart. Mustard prefers heavy feeding: Regularly add well-rotted manure or compost to the soil. Mustard supposedly stimulates growth of beans, grapes, and fruit trees. It is said to keep flea beetles away from collards. Mustard also releases a chemical in the soil that inhibits cyst nematodes and prevents root rot and also many other plants from growing near it.

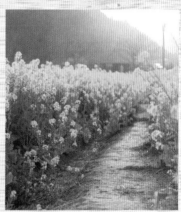

To grow mustard for its leaves, sow seeds at several intervals from spring through early fall. If you're growing mustard for its seeds, sow in spring or late summer. Once established, it will easily self-sow; it can even become a garden pest.

Harvest leaves for salads when they are young and tender. Harvest seeds when pods have turned brown but before they split open. Spread plants on a tray. Within a couple of weeks the seeds should ripen. Store whole or ground mustard seed in tightly covered jars.

Health Benefits

Mustard has many medicinal uses, too. If you're old enough, you may even remember getting a mustard plaster when you had a cold. Mustard seeds warm the skin and open the lungs to make breathing easier. Mustard plasters may also relieve rheumatism, toothache, sore muscles, and arthritis.

Mustard is loaded with antimicrobial and anti-inflammatory properties, many of which can be inhaled through the vapors.

In folk medicine some herbs have been labeled "counterirritants." These herbs stimulate blood flow to the skin and the muscles underneath. Practically speaking, counterirritants encourage healing and provide pain relief for those aching muscles. Two commonly used counterirritants in folk healing are cayenne pepper and mustard seeds. This simple mustard plaster can be used when your muscles ache:

Crush the seeds of white or brown mustard. Moisten with vinegar and sprinkle with flour. Spread mixture on a cloth, and cover with a second cloth. Lay the moist side on the painful area, and leave on for 20 minutes. (Remove the plaster if it becomes painful.)

Home Remedies

A cup of hot tea with honey loosens up your nasal passages and makes that stuffy nose feel better. Folk healers have known this secret for centuries. They often suggest drinking tea with spices and herbs that contain aromatic oils with antiviral properties, including mustard.

Mustard seed has sulfur-containing compounds that stimulate the flow of mucus. To get the full effect of the expectorant compounds, the mustard seeds must be broken and allowed to sit in water for 15 minutes. Crush 1 teaspoon mustard seeds or grind them in a coffee grinder. Place the seeds in a cup of warm water. Steep for 15 minutes. This concoction might be a little hard to swallow, so take it in 1/4-cup doses throughout the day.

A tablespoon or two of powdered mustard in a basin of nice warm water can relieve cramps caused by PMS, but don't drink it. Soak your feet in it to reap the relaxing effects.

Impress Grandma by making a mustard plaster. Here are three options:

1. For chest colds, mix 1 tablespoon dry mustard and 2 to 4 tablespoons flour. Mix both with 1 egg white (optional) and warm water to form a paste. Next, find a clean handkerchief or square of muslin large enough to cover the upper chest. Smear the cloth the same way you'd smear mustard on a sandwich, then plop another cloth over it. Dab olive oil on the patient's skin and apply the mustard plaster to the upper chest. Check yourself or the patient every few minutes since mustard plaster can burn. Remove after a few minutes. Afterward, wash off any traces of mustard from the skin.

2. For aches caused by gout, mix 1 part mustard powder (or crushed mustard seeds) to 1 part whole wheat flour and add enough water to form a thick paste. Slather petroleum jelly, vegetable shortening, or lard on the affected area. Spread a thick coat of mustard paste on a piece of gauze or cloth, then apply over the greased-up area. Tape down and leave in place for several hours or overnight.

3. To make a poultice, mix powdered seeds with an equal amount of flour and enough water to form a paste. Spread mustard plaster on a cloth and place the cloth, poultice side down, on the skin. Leave on about 20 minutes. Remove if the poultice becomes uncomfortable. Wash affected area.

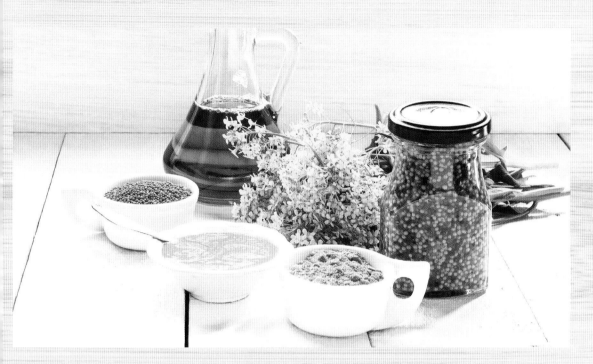

Ideas for Use

Its chief constituent, mustard oil, gives it its heat and flavor. These constituents also make mustard an appetite stimulate and a powerful irritant. Mustard in small doses improves digestion. Young leaves are vitamin-rich additions to salads, or they can be boiled with onions and salt pork.

Cautions

Consuming large quantities of mustard seed may cause vomiting. Don't leave mustard plasters on too long or they may blister skin.

Make Your Own

You haven't really tasted mustard until you've made it yourself. To make mustard from seeds, boil ⅓ cup cider vinegar, ⅔ cup cider, 2 tablespoons honey, ⅛ tablespoon turmeric, and up to 1 teaspoon salt. While hot, combine with ¼ cup ground mustard seeds. Blend in a food processor. After the mixture is smooth, add 1 tablespoon olive oil. This recipe makes 1 ¼ cups of mustard. Another recipe is found on the following page.

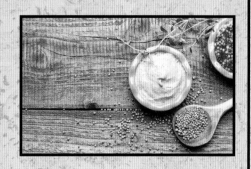

Hot & Spicy Mustard

- ¼ cup water
- ¼ cup whole yellow mustard seeds
- ¼ cup honey
- 3 tablespoons cider vinegar
- 2 tablespoons ground mustard
- 1 teaspoon salt
- ⅛ teaspoon ground cloves

1. Place water in small saucepan. Bring to a boil over high heat. Add mustard seeds. Cover saucepan; remove from heat. Let stand 1 hour or until liquid is absorbed.

2. Combine mustard seeds, honey, vinegar, ground mustard, salt and cloves in food processor; process using on/off pulsing action until mixture is thickened and seeds are coarsely chopped, scraping down side of work bowl once. Refrigerate at least 1 day before serving. Store in airtight container in refrigerator up to 3 weeks.

Makes about 1 cup

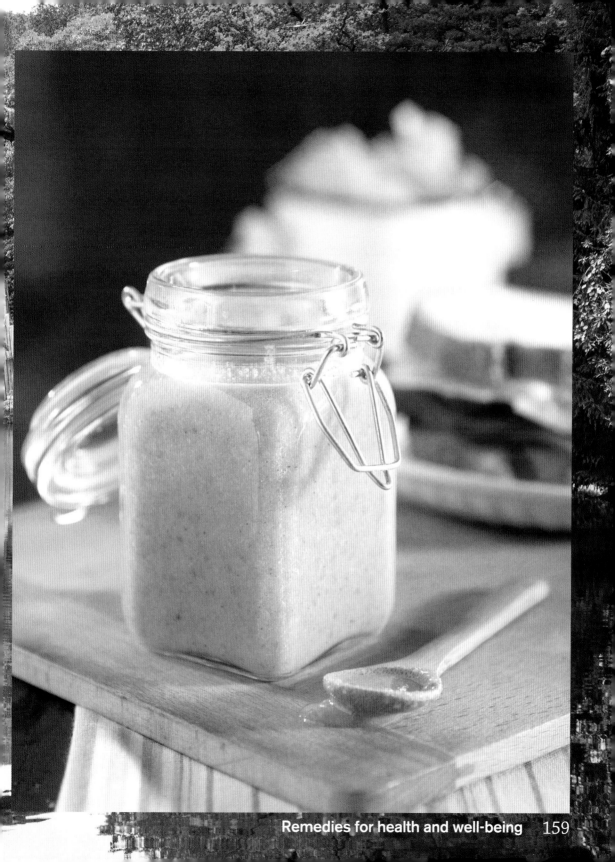

Nutmeg and Mace

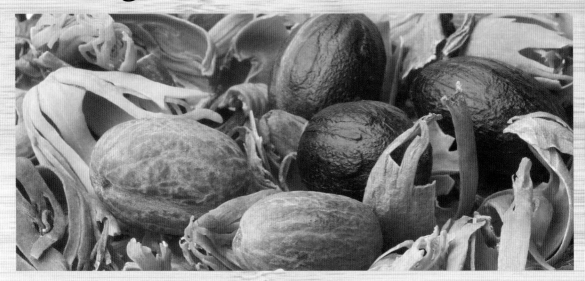

The nutmeg tree, an evergreen plant, actually produces two spices: nutmeg from the tree's seed and mace from the seed covering. They're both slightly sweet and have a delightful smell. Both are used to flavor baked goods and other foods. Mace is also used to help preserve food.

The Plant

The tree originates in the Banda Islands of Indonesia—commonly known as the Spice Islands. Today, it's also grown in Caribbean regions. It became popular in Europe during the middle ages and saw its popularity spike during the Elizabethan Era—not for its taste, but because it was seen as something that could ward of the plague. Nutmeg trees can grow quite tall, up to 65 feet. When the fruit is mature, people can harvest the nutmeg and its surrounding covering, the mace.

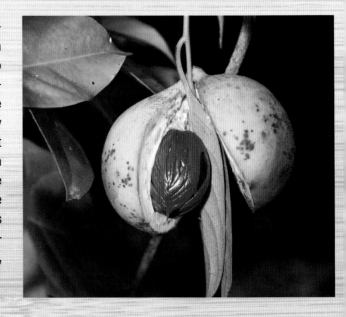

Health Benefits and Folk Remedies

There's no real scientific evidence for the use of nutmeg to heal in humans, though one 2016 study did examine the use of nutmeg oil as an anti-inflammatory and pain reliever for rats and concluded that nutmeg oil could potentially help chronic inflammation. An earlier animal study in 2009 examined the use of the oil as an anticonvulsant and did show promising results in preventing seizure spread. One of nutmeg's compounds, called myristicin, is a psychoactive drug that can cause various negative effects, including palpitations and anxiety.

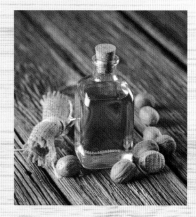

In folk medicine, nutmeg has been used internally as a remedy for diarrhea, nausea, and gas, and topically to help aches and toothache.

Steep a tea with 1 teaspoon cumin seeds and a pinch of nutmeg to soothe tummy troubles.

For insomnia, soak 10 raw almonds overnight in water to soften, then peel off the skins. Put almonds in blender with 1 cup warm milk, a pinch of ginger, and a pinch of nutmeg. Drink at night to relax you before going to bed. Or just put a pinch of nutmeg in warm milk.

Nutmeg Butter

The oil of the nutmeg can be expressed as a substance called nutmeg butter, which is edible but can also be used to provide fragrance to soaps and perfumes.

Ideas for Use

Nutmeg can be used in both sweet and savory dishes—and, of course, eggnog!

Cautions

Don't eat in large quantities for risk of hallucinations and psychoactive effects. Nutmeg and mace should also be treated with caution if taken with certain liver medications. Large quantities should not be taken during pregnancy. Large quantities may be toxic to children and pets especially.

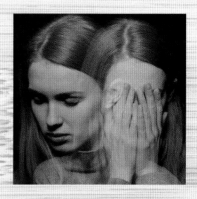

Honey Fig Whole Wheat Muffins

- 1 cup whole wheat flour
- ½ cup all-purpose flour
- ½ cup wheat germ
- 2 teaspoons baking powder
- 1 teaspoon ground cinnamon
- ½ teaspoon salt
- ½ teaspoon ground nutmeg
- ½ cup milk
- ½ cup honey
- ¼ cup (1/2 stick) butter, melted
- 1 egg
- 1 cup chopped dried figs
- ½ cup chopped walnuts

1. Preheat oven to 375°F. Grease 12 standard (2½-inch) muffin cups or line with paper baking cups.

2. Combine flours, wheat germ, baking powder, cinnamon, salt and nutmeg in large bowl. Combine milk, honey, butter and egg in small bowl until well blended. Stir into flour mixture just until moistened. Fold in figs and walnuts. Spoon evenly into prepared muffin cups.

3. Bake 20 minutes or until lightly browned on edges and toothpick inserted in center comes out clean. Remove from pan.

Makes 12 muffins

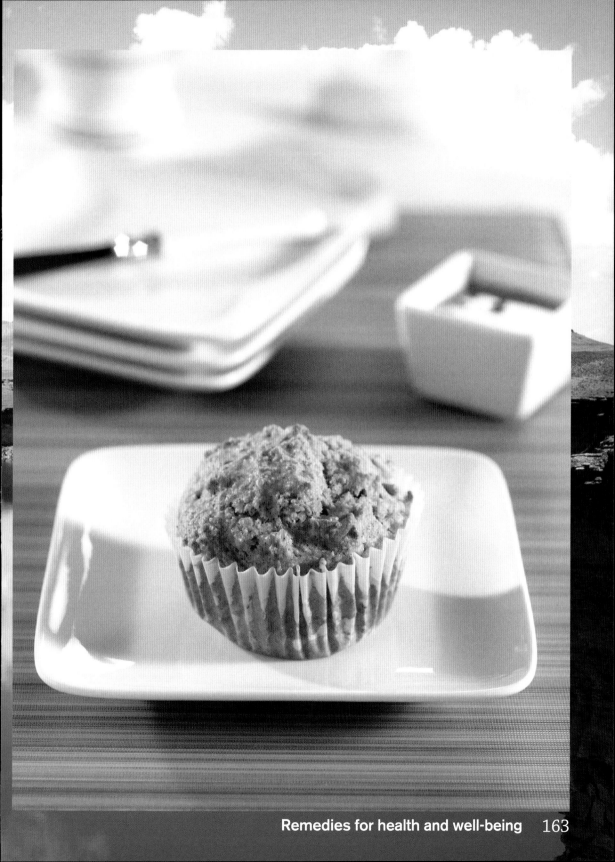

Paprika

As seasoning, paprika adds color and flavor to a variety of dishes. For those seeking to lower their blood pressure by lowering their salt intake, paprika is one of the three essential "P's" to start with, along with parsley and pepper.

A Versatile Spice

The spice originated in South America, although today it's associated strongly with Hungarian cuisine in the national dish goulash and, of course, paprikash. Derived from mild peppers, paprika comes in a variety of flavors depending on what peppers were used in its creation—it can be mild or pungency, sweet or spicy. Sweet, hot, and smoked paprika all exist. Hungary is a main producer of paprika, producing eight different kinds, while Spanish paprika comes in several varieties as well.

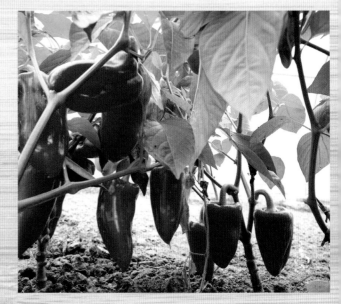

Colorful and Healthy

TThe bright color of paprika comes from its carotenoids, with different carotenoids present based on the originating pepper. One study noted that red paprika is generally highest in a carotenoid called capsanthin, while orange paprika is higher in zeaxanthin, one of the antioxidant carotenoids that has links to eye health. Beta-carotene helps provide yellow or orange color to paprika. Foods high in carotenoids are believed to have a protective effect against various forms of cancer. Carotenoids also play a role in keeping your skin and eyes healthy, as beta-carotene is converted into vitamin A in your body. Amazingly, one tablespoon of paprika contains 70 percent of your daily value (DV) of vitamin A, crucial for good vision and general immune health.

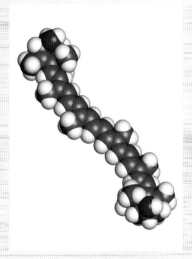

Paprika also contains smaller but significant amounts of a number of vitamins and minerals. For instance, it contains 10 percent of your DV of vitamin E, an antioxidant that protects against cell damage, diseases of the brain and nervous system. It contains 8 percent of your DV of vitamin C, necessary for healing and forming muscle and cartilage. It contains 14 percent of your DV of vitamin B6, a vitamin that is needed for any number of bodily functions involved in body development and metabolism. The iron in paprika amounts to 9 percent of the DV, so it helps prevent anemia. The spice also contains smaller amounts of vitamin K, riboflavin, niacin, and potassium.

Ideas for Use

A sprinkle of paprika can add visual interest to a macaroni or potato salad or devilled eggs. Paprika will add a burst of flavor to scrambled eggs, yogurt, and hummus, and you can also make your own salad dressings that include it as one of the spices. It adds great flavor to chicken, potatoes, and legumes. Roasted chickpeas and other roasted vegetables perk up with the addition of paprika.

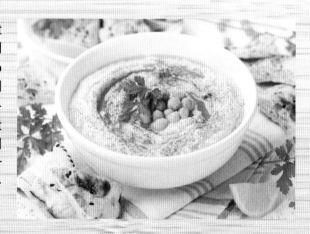

Spanish Braised Chicken with Green Olives & Rice

- 2 pounds bone-in skinless chicken thighs
- 1 teaspoon paprika
- ¾ cup dry sherry
- 2¼ cups water
- 1 can (about 14 ounces) fat-free reduced-sodium chicken broth
- ¾ cup sliced pimiento-stuffed green olives
- 1½ teaspoons dried sage
- 1½ cups uncooked long grain white rice

1. Sprinkle chicken thighs with paprika. Spray large nonstick skillet with nonstick cooking spray; heat over medium-high heat. Cook chicken 6 to 8 minutes or until browned on both sides, turning once.

2. Remove chicken from skillet. Add sherry, stirring to scrape up brown bits from bottom of skillet. Add water, broth, olives and sage; bring to a boil. Reduce heat to low. Return chicken to skillet. Cover and simmer 10 minutes.

3. Add rice to liquid around chicken; gently stir to distribute evenly in skillet. Cover; simmer 20 to 25 minutes or until rice is tender and chicken is cooked through (165°F).

Makes 6 servings

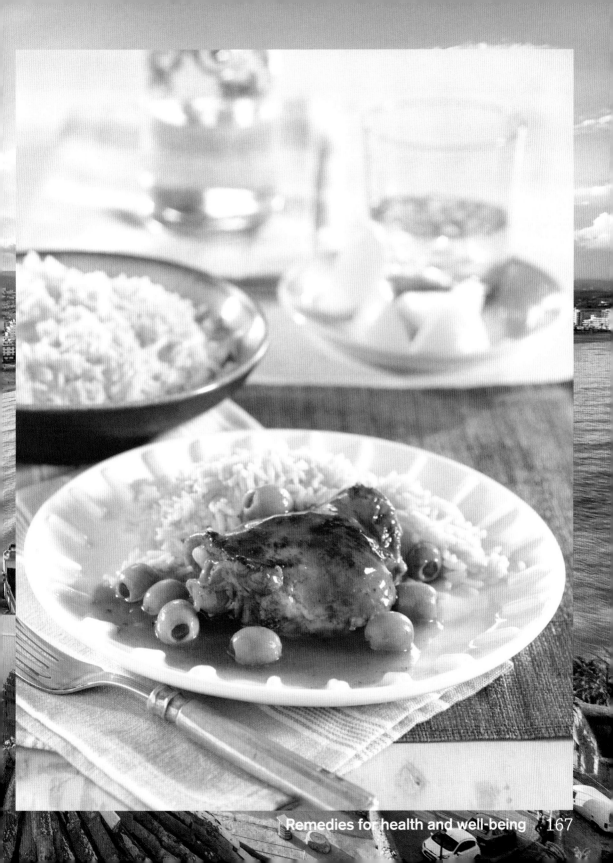

Poppy Seed

You may have heard that consuming poppy seeds before a drug test can result in a false positive. And surprisingly, this is true. In fact, many government agencies that run frequent random drug tests encourage their employees to avoid ingesting the tiny seeds. And inmates in federal prisons are prohibited from eating poppy seeds, even when granted temporary furlough.

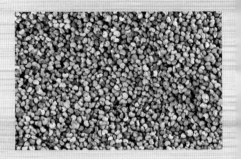

Fortunately, even though poppy seeds come from the same plant—the opium poppy—that is used to make heroin and morphine, these small kidney-shaped seeds are far more beneficial than they are dangerous. In fact, although eating poppy seeds may expose you to trace amounts of opiates, you would have to eat huge amounts of these tiny seeds to feel any sort of psychological effects such as those you would feel from heroin or morphine.

About the Poppy

Poppy seeds are obtained from the *Papaver somniferum*, a flowering plant which is often called the breadseed poppy—a much less nefarious-sounding name than its other common name, the opium poppy. As the name suggests, the seeds of the breadseed poppy are edible, and are often used as an ingredient in pastries and bread. They can also be pressed to produce an oil, which is used for cooking, as a lamp oil, in paints, and in soap. Poppy seeds are mostly cultivated in Central Europe, with almost a third of the world's supply coming from the Czech Republic.

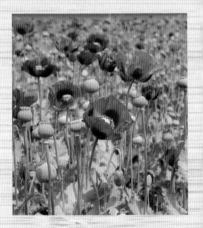

Packed with Benefits

The oil and seeds of the *Papaver somniferum* are mentioned in medical texts dating back thousands of years, when the Egyptians, Greeks, and Romans would use the seeds for digestive disorders, as a sedative, or for respiratory issues. Today, we know that poppy seeds have a great nutritional profile, containing protein and fiber as well as high amounts of several vitamins and minerals, including manganese, calcium, iron, zinc, and magnesium. Poppy seeds are also high in linoleic acid, an omega-6 fatty acid, which, when eaten in moderation, can protect against heart disease.

Health Benefits

The minerals and nutrients in poppy seeds help to protect against a host of issues. Fiber aids digestion, helping to prevent or treat constipation. Iron prevents anemia, increases blood flow, and improves cognitive performance. Calcium and manganese strengthen bones and connective tissues. And zinc helps to boost the immune system, warding off respiratory infections and aiding the production of immune cells in the body. One study even shows that poppy seeds have potential as a cancer treatment. The seeds increase the activity of an enzyme called "glutathione-S-transferase," which has the ability to neutralize carcinogens. The study proved that poppy seeds increased the effectiveness of this enzyme by an impressive 78 percent in the stomach, liver, and esophagus.

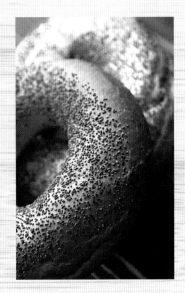

Not Just Edible

These tiny seeds don't need to be ingested to obtain some of their benefits; the nutrients in poppy seeds are great for skin health, as well. Poppy seeds can be soaked in water or milk and then ground into a paste, which can be applied to the skin to relieve burns, itching, and inflammation. This paste also works well as a moisturizer, especially with the addition of honey. Simply apply the mixture to skin, let it sit for about 10 minutes, then rinse off.

Ideas for Use

Poppy seeds can be found in most grocery and health food stores, often in the bulk bins, and there are a variety of ways to use them. When they are raw they have little taste, but roasting them brings out their nutty flavor. The seeds are perfect for sprinkling over oatmeal or yogurt to add some crunch, or mixing into a homemade granola recipe. And of course, poppy seeds are delicious in breads, cakes, muffins, and pastries. The seeds can also be ground in a blender or coffee grinder to create a gluten-free "flour" that can be used in baking.

Cautions

While most people have no problems eating the amounts of poppy seeds found in food, talk to a doctor if you plan on eating larger quantities. And steer clear of "poppy tea," which is sometimes made with large enough quantities of the seeds to have negative side effects.

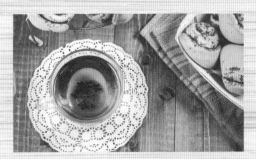

Strawberry Poppy Seed Chicken Salad

Dressing

- ¼ cup white wine vinegar
- 2 tablespoons orange juice
- 1 tablespoon sugar
- 2 teaspoons poppy seeds
- 1½ teaspoons Dijon mustard
- ½ teaspoon salt
- ½ teaspoon minced dried onion
- ½ cup vegetable oil

Salad

- 8 cups romaine lettuce
- 1 package (12 to 16 ounces) grilled or roasted chicken breast strips
- ¾ cup fresh pineapple chunks
- ¾ cup sliced fresh strawberries
- ¾ cup fresh blueberries
- 1 navel orange, peeled and sectioned or 1 can (11 ounces) mandarin oranges, drained
- ¼ cup chopped toasted pecans

1. For dressing, combine vinegar, orange juice, sugar, poppy seeds, mustard, salt and dried onion in small bowl; mix well. Slowly add oil, whisking until well blended.

2. For salad, combine romaine and two thirds of dressing in large bowl; toss gently to coat. Divide salad among 4 plates, top with chicken, pineapple, strawberries, blueberries, oranges and pecans. Serve with remaining dressing.

Makes 4 servings

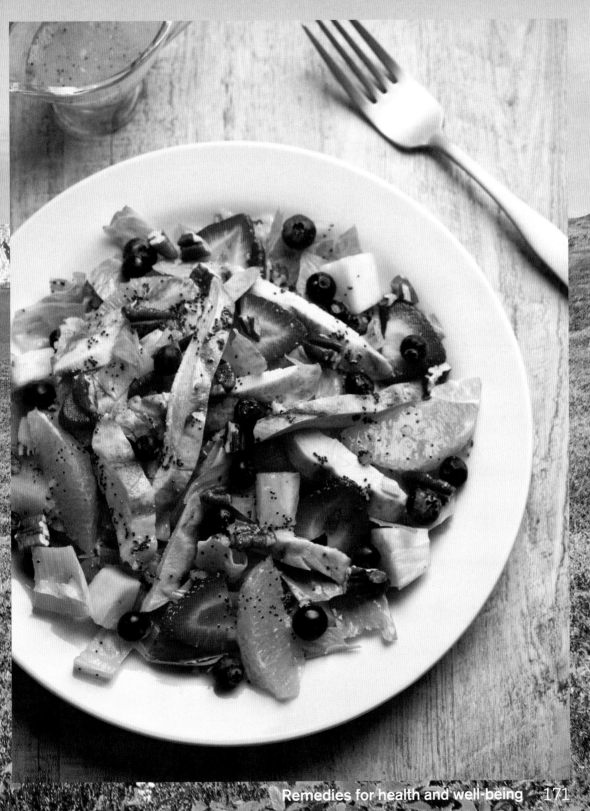

Saffron

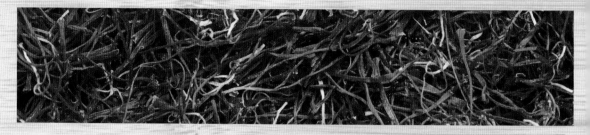

Derived from the perennial flower *Crocus sativus*, saffron is one of the world's most expensive spices. A pound of these vividly hued threads can cost up to $5,000. While that may seem excessive, producing this coveted spice requires an immense amount of work. The saffron itself is the long, spindly stigma inside the *Crocus sativus*, and each flower averages about 7 milligrams of dried spice. The flowers only bloom for one to two weeks in the middle of autumn, and to obtain a pound of dried saffron, workers must harvest around 75,000 flowers. The job is complicated by the fact that the flowers must be picked as soon as they bloom, because they wilt within a day. The limited blooming time and hasty harvest mean that this spice is not only expensive, but also rare.

History

The *Crocus sativus* probably originated in Iran, Greece, or Mesopotamia, and eventually made its way throughout Asia and Europe before finding its way to Northern Africa, North America and the Pacific islands. Today, the flower is grown on every continent except Antarctica, but Iran is the largest producer of saffron, responsible for around 90 percent of the world's supply. With its distinctive yellow-orange color, saffron has been used as a pigment and dye for at least 50,000 years. But there is evidence that many ancient cultures also used the spice medicinally. Egyptian and Roman healers prescribed it for digestive disorders and respiratory illnesses, while Persians used the spice to make tea to cure melancholy. And Alexander the Great was believed to have made use of saffron, infusing his bathwater with the spice as a remedy for battle wounds.

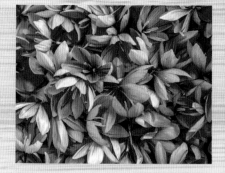

Saffron has been so prized throughout history that it even sparked a war in the 14th century, when demand for the spice skyrocketed during the Black Plague. Large amounts of the spice were shipped to Europe to be used for medications, but one shipment was stolen by nobles. The ensuing uproar amongst the people was known as the Saffron War, and resulted in new cultivation of the spice throughout Europe.

172   Turmeric & Healing Spices

Health Benefits

One look at the many benefits saffron has to offer, and it's clear to see why this spice has been grown and sought after—not to mention fought over—for centuries. Saffron has many compounds that act as antioxidants, including crocin and crocetin, the pigments responsible for its bright color. These compounds help to prevent inflammation and neutralize free radicals, and may even hold the key to future cancer treatments. In fact, lab studies have shown that the compounds in saffron can isolate and kill cancer cells, while leaving healthy cells unharmed. While more research on human subjects is needed, the findings are extremely promising. And it turns out that the Persians were on to something when they drank saffron tea for "melancholy." Several studies have shown that taking 30 milligrams of saffron daily is just as effective as prescription medication for relieving depression. Another study found that simply smelling saffron for 20 minutes was effective at reducing anxiety and the stress hormone cortisol. It's no wonder that saffron is often nicknamed "the sunshine spice"!

Research has also shown that saffron may help to curb appetite, aiding weight loss or preventing weight gain. In one study, one group of women took saffron supplements, while another group was given a placebo. After eight weeks, the group taking the saffron reported snacking less often and had lost more weight than the placebo group. Another study showed that participants taking saffron supplements lowered their body mass index and waist circumference. Scientists are unsure of how saffron suppresses appetite, although they theorize it may be linked to the spice's mood-elevating benefits.

Ideas for Use

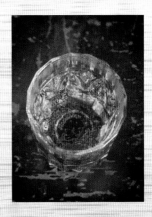

Saffron is readily available in many stores and most specialty markets. Although it's expensive, a very small amount of the spice goes a long way. To draw out the flavor, soak the saffron threads in hot water, then add the liquid to your recipe. Try a pinch of the spice in rice dishes, such as paella or risotto, or in vegetables, meat, seafood, or poultry. It can even be used in sweet desserts, like rice pudding or pastries. The threads can also be used to make tea, often simmered with ginger, cinnamon, and honey to create a comforting and mood-lifting beverage.

Cautions

While the high cost of saffron makes it unlikely that you'll ever have more than a gram or two on hand, it should be noted that large doses of the spice (more than one and a half grams per day) are extremely unsafe and can cause poisoning. But the small amounts found in food or supplements have proven their worth, earning a spot in the kitchen spice rack.

Risotto alla Milanese

- ¼ teaspoon saffron threads
- 3½ to 4 cups chicken broth
- 4 tablespoons butter, divided
- 1 large onion, chopped
- 1½ cups uncooked arborio or short-grain white rice
- ½ cup dry white wine
- ½ teaspoon salt
- ¼ cup grated Parmesan cheese
  Dash black pepper

*** Chopped fresh parsley (optional)

1. Crush saffron to a powder; place in glass measuring cup.

2. Bring broth to a boil in medium saucepan over medium heat; reduce heat to low. Stir ½ cup broth into saffron to dissolve; set aside. Keep remaining broth hot.

3. Heat 3 tablespoons butter in large saucepan over medium heat until melted and bubbly. Add onion; cook and stir 5 minutes or until onion is soft. Add rice; cook and stir 2 minutes. Stir in wine, salt and pepper; cook over medium-high heat 3 to 5 minutes until wine is absorbed, stirring occasionally.

4. Reduce heat to medium-low. Stir ½ cup hot broth into rice mixture; cook and stir until broth is absorbed. Repeat, adding ½ up broth three more times, cooking and stirring until broth is absorbed.

5. Add saffron-flavored broth to rice; cook until absorbed. Continue to add remaining broth, ½ cup at a time, cooking and stirring until rice is tender but firm and mixture has slight creamy consistency. (Not all broth may be necessary. Total cooking time will be 20 to 25 minutes.)

6. Remove risotto from heat. Stir in remaining 1 tablespoon butter and cheese. Sprinkle with parsley, if desired. Serve immediately.

Makes 6 to 8 servings

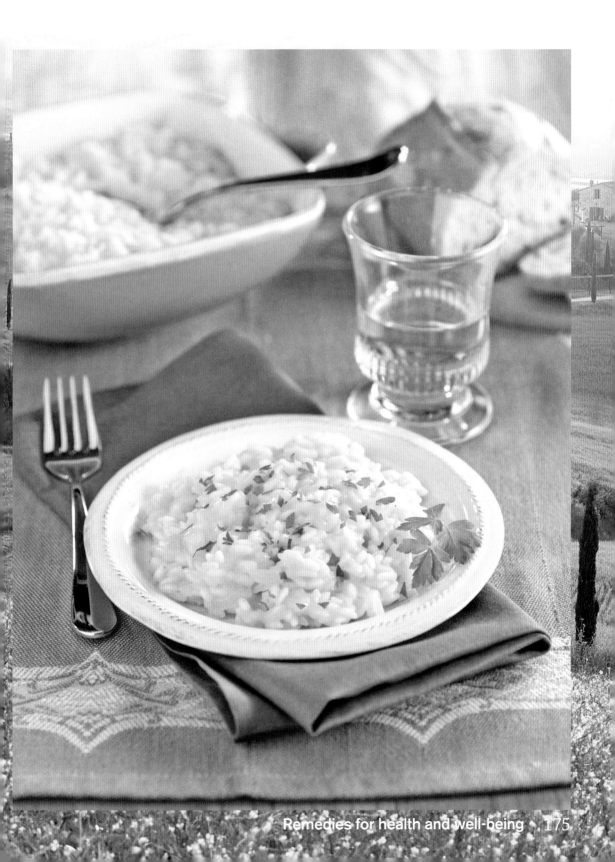

Sesame Seed

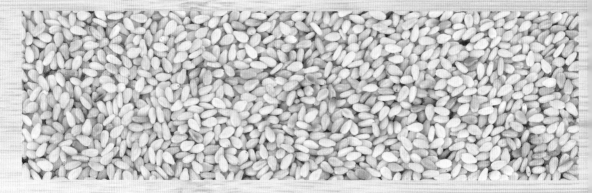

The sesame plant was domesticated more than 3,000 years ago, maybe as long as 5,000 years ago, in what is now India. While wild sesame still grows in some areas, domestic sesame grows in numerous tropical regions.

With their gold mine of healthy minerals and their niacin and folic-acid contents, seeds are an excellent nutrition package. They are among the better plant sources of iron and zinc. And they provide more fiber per ounce than nuts. They are also good sources of protein. Sesame seeds in particular are a surprising source of the bone-building mineral calcium, great news for folks who have trouble tolerating dairy products. And seeds in general are a rich source of vitamin E. The only drawback: Some seeds are quite high in fat. Sesame seeds provide about 80 percent of their calories as fat, although the fat is mostly of the heart-smart unsaturated variety.

The Plant

The plant grows to a height of 1.6 to 3.3 feet tall, and has tubular flowers that come in varying colors. The seeds, too, come in different colors and sizes. A drought-tolerate plant, sesame is grown in warm areas. Tanzania and India are large producers and exporters of the crop; Japan is the larger importer, as sesame oil is used extensively in Japanese cooking. The pods split open naturally when the seeds are ripe; one theory for the origin of the phrase "Open, sesame," from the story of Ali Baba and the Forty Thieves is that it refers to how sesame pods open to reveal the treasure of sesame seeds.

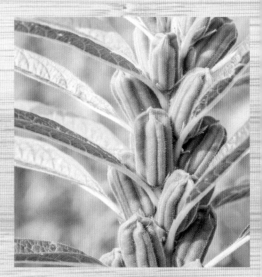

Nutritional Powerhouses

Nutritionally, sesame seeds are a treasure. A quarter cup of dried sesame seeds can provide the daily recommended intake of copper, and substantial amounts of manganese, calcium, phosphorous, magnesium, iron, zinc, and vitamin B1. A serving provides more than 6 grams of protein and 4 grams of fiber.

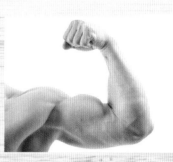

Health Benefits

Sesame seeds have a high phytosterol content, a substance believed to lower cholesterol. They also contain substances called sesamin and sesmolin that are believed to lower cholesterol.

Sesame seeds, along with pumpkins and sunflower seeds, are packed with essential fatty acids necessary for brain function.

Sesame seeds may help if you're suffering from constipation. They provide roughage and bulk, and they soften the contents of the intestines, which makes elimination easier. Eat no more than ½ ounce daily, and drink lots of water as you take the seeds. You may also sprinkle them on salads and other foods, but again, no more than ½ ounce.

Because sesame seeds are rich in omega-6 fatty acid, which may be missing in women who suffer with PMS, they may be able to ease PMS symptoms.

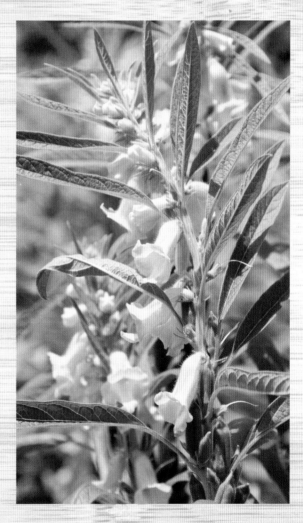

Sesame Oil

Sesame seed oil may help lower blood cholesterol level when taken in place of saturated fats.

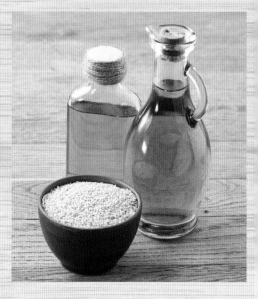

Dry nasal passages are prime breeding grounds for the cold virus. Although doctors typically recommend saline nose drops during the winter to keep nasal passages moist, one study compared saline drops to sesame oil. The people who used sesame oil had an 80 percent improvement in their nasal dryness while the people who used traditional saline drops had a 30 percent improvement. While it may not be a good idea to shoot sesame oil up your nose (it could get into the lungs), try rubbing a drop around the inside of your nostrils.

Anecdotally, depression associated with Alzheimer's disease may be relieved with nose drops of warmed sesame oil. Use about 3 drops per nostril, twice a day. Some say you can also help relieve depression by rubbing a little of that warmed sesame oil on the top of the head and bottoms of the feet.

Gargling with warm sesame oil is an Ayurvedic treatment for gum disease. Take a mouthful and swish it around twice a day, then rinse. It's also said that this simple gargle can reduce cheek wrinkles. What a great bonus!

For a nice relaxation technique if you're suffering from stress or insomnia, warm a few ounces of sesame oil and rub it all over your body, from head to toe. Sunflower and corn oil work well, too. After your massage, take a long, hot soak in the tub.

Ideas for Use

Toasted sesame seeds are a great addition to oil-based salad dressing. They can add a crunch when put in baked goods. They make a great addition to vegetable stir fries. Sesame is also available in a butter or paste and in Middle Eastern dips, such as tahini. And sesame paste can be a chief ingredient in halva, a popular Middle Eastern and Mediterranean desert (halva may also be based on sunflower paste).

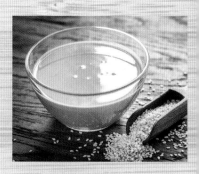

Cautions

Make sure sesame seeds are stored in an airtight container in a dry space or they can become rancid.

If you have diverticulosis, consult your doctor about what seeds and nuts you should eat or avoid. The age-old advice for people with diverticulosis was to avoid all nuts, seeds, and hulls. It is now recommended that only foods that are sharp, hard, or large enough to irritate or get caught in the diverticula be avoided. These include nuts, popcorn hulls, and sunflower, pumpkin, caraway, and sesame seeds.

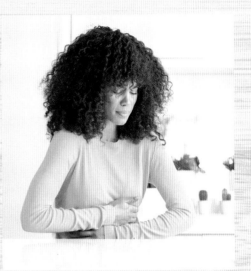

Sensational Seeds

While you're picking up seeds in the supermarket, check out some of these other seeds.

Sunflower seeds contain more than 80 percent of your daily recommended intake of vitamin E, which provides anti-inflammatory and cardiovascular benefits. Vitamin E is also believed to protect brain health. Sunflowers seeds are also rich in copper, vitamin B1, selenium, phosphorous, manganese, vitamin B6, and magnesium.

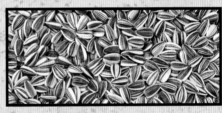

Pumpkin seeds are rich in manganese, phosphorous, copper, magnesium, and zinc—though if you're eating for the zinc, eat the unshelled versions. Pumpkin seeds are rich in antioxidants, which may help reduce cancer risk. They also provide a boost of protein, with more than 9 grams found in a serving.

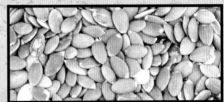

Hemp seeds—you may see them marketed as "hemp heart"—are also rich in protein, with 11 grams in a serving. They're rich in iron, magnesium, and zinc. And no, while hemp seeds are grown from the same plant that makes marijuana, they do not contain THC, so you will not get a high if you sprinkle them on your salad or into your yogurt.

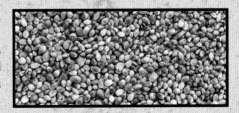

Roast Sesame Fish

- 4 skinless tilapia fillets (about 5 ounces each)
- ¼ cup plus 1 tablespoon tamari or soy sauce, divided
- 1 teaspoon dark sesame oil, divided
- 2 teaspoons sesame seeds
- 2 tablespoons sake or dry sherry
- 2 to 3 teaspoons grated fresh ginger
- 1 teaspoon sugar

*** 1 teaspoon wasabi paste (optional)

1. Preheat oven to 400°F. Place fish in shallow baking dish. Combine 1 tablespoon tamari and ½ teaspoon sesame oil in small bowl; brush over fish. Sprinkle sesame seeds over fish. Bake 10 to 15 minutes or until fish is opaque in center.

2. Meanwhile, combine remaining ¼ cup tamari, ½ teaspoon sesame oil, sake, ginger, sugar and wasabi paste, if desired, in small bowl. Drizzle sauce over fish before serving.

Makes 4 servings

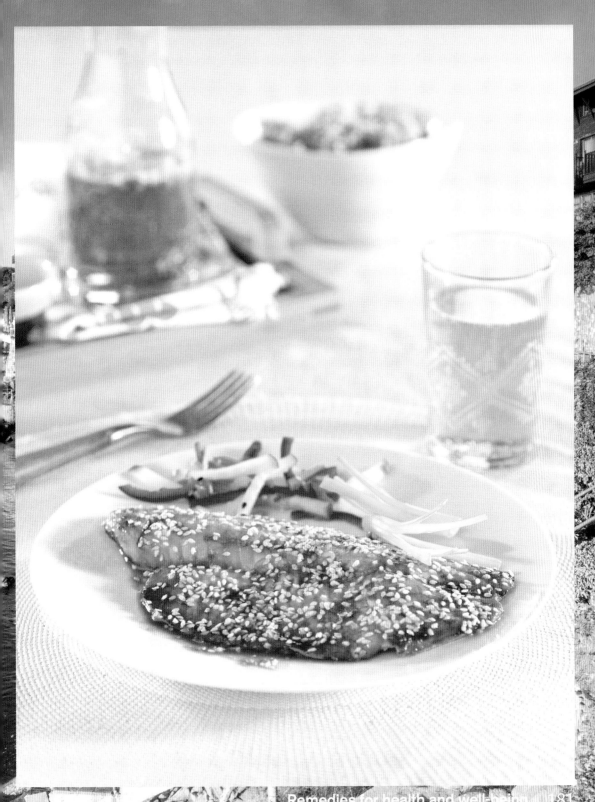

Star Anise

If you've ever suffered from a bout with the flu, star anise is one spice you'll want to know about. This flower-shaped fruit, which is harvested from the *Illicium verum* evergreen tree, has natural antiviral properties thanks to a compound called shikimic acid. In fact, this compound is used to create the medication oseltamivir—better known as Tamiflu. But warding off the flu is only one of many benefits this sweet spice possesses.

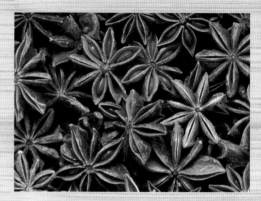

About the Plant

The *Illicium verum* tree is native to Vietnam and China. The star-shaped fruits of the tree are picked before they're ripe and dried in the sun until they harden, producing distinct reddish-orange pods. The flavor of star anise is often described as licorice-like, and is very similar to anise seed, although the two spices are surprisingly unrelated. The spice has been a popular ingredient in China for centuries, where it is also prized as a medicinal remedy. Today, most star anise is produced in China and Japan, but it is used all over the world.

Many Uses

Star anise is a popular spice in many Asian cuisines, including biryani, a rice dish served in India, and pho, a Vietnamese noodle soup. The spice is also common in flavorful masala chai tea and is one of the five spices included in traditional Chinese five-spice seasoning. Its distinct flavor and sweet scent make star anise a versatile ingredient for many non-food items, as well. The spice is often used in mouthwash, skin cream, toothpaste, perfumes, and cosmetics. But the vast majority of the world's supply—around 90 percent—is used to create antiviral medications.

Flu Fighter

In addition to shikimic acid, star anise contains several other beneficial compounds, including linalool, quercetin, anethole, and vitamin C. Together, these compounds give the spice antioxidant, anti-inflammatory, and antimicrobial properties, providing it with a range of medicinal benefits. Star anise's claim to fame is its flu-fighting ability. And while Tamiflu is commonly prescribed for those who have been knocked down with the illness, a cup of star anise tea may be even more effective. Studies have shown that the combination of shikimic acid and quercetin in the spice increases the production of immune cells even more than Tamiflu alone.

Bacteria Buster

Star anise has also been shown to prevent the growth of bacteria, with studies demonstrating that the spice inhibits the common *E. coli* bacteria, responsible for gastrointestinal infections and pneumonia, as well as dozens of different antibiotic-resistant strains of bacteria. Research suggests that the spice may also be effective at warding off fungal infections. While most of these studies have been limited to animal and test tube research, the findings are encouraging for scientists in search of future treatments.

Other Health Benefits

With its abundant antioxidants, star anise may help to support a healthy heart. Some studies have shown that the spice helps to regulate weight and blood pressure, while reducing the amount of plaque in the arteries. And the compound anethole in the spice has been found to be beneficial for maintaining a healthy blood sugar level. There is even evidence that star anise may be effective at preventing cancer, by increasing certain enzymes that inhibit the disease.

Ideas for Use

Star anise is not only versatile when it comes to health benefits, but it's also versatile when it comes to cuisine, giving you numerous ways to sample the sweet spice. It's easy to incorporate into recipes, pairing well with coriander, cinnamon, clove, and cardamom, and balancing out savory dishes. The dried pods can be ground and added to Chinese-inspired recipes or mixed into baked goods, or the whole pods can be simmered in stews, soups, or broths to add depth of flavor. Or, take a page from traditional Chinese medicine and steep the pods in hot water to make a soothing (and flu-fighting!) tea.

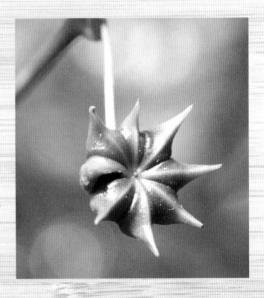

Cautions

Finally, be sure to check the source of your star anise to confirm that it is derived from the Chinese *Illicium verum* tree. Japanese star anise—derived from the similar *Illicium anisatum*—is highly toxic and inedible. While the FDA monitors imports of star anise to be sure the Japanese type is not sold as food, always purchase the spice from a reputable company.

Red Cooked Pork Roast

- 1 tablespoon peanut or canola oil
- 3 to 3½ pounds boneless pork shoulder roast (pork butt)
- ½ cup chicken broth
- ¼ cup soy sauce
- 4 cloves garlic, minced
- 3 whole star anise
- 1 tablespoon water
- 1 tablespoon cornstarch
- 4 drops red food coloring

*** Hot cooked Chinese noodles or rice

1. Heat oil in Dutch oven or large deep ovenproof skillet with lid over medium heat until hot. Add pork; cook until browned, 6 to 7 minutes per side.

2. Meanwhile, preheat oven to 325°F. Combine broth, soy sauce, garlic and star anise in small bowl; pour over pork in Dutch oven. Cover and bake 3 hours or until pork is very tender when pierced with fork. Transfer to cutting board; tent with foil.

3. Discard star anise; skim off and discard fat from pan juices. Stir water into cornstarch in small bowl; mix well. Place Dutch oven with pan juices over medium heat; stir in cornstarch mixture. Bring to a boil, stirring constantly. Simmer 2 to 3 minutes or until sauce thickens. Stir in food coloring.

4. Cut meat into chunks (or shred); return to Dutch oven to toss with sauce and heat through. Serve with noodles.

Makes 6 to 8 servings

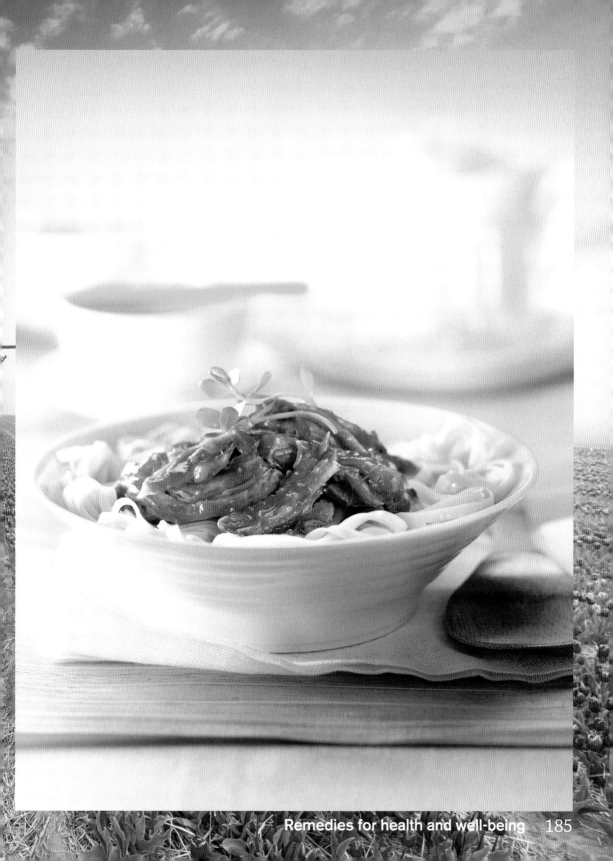

Sumac

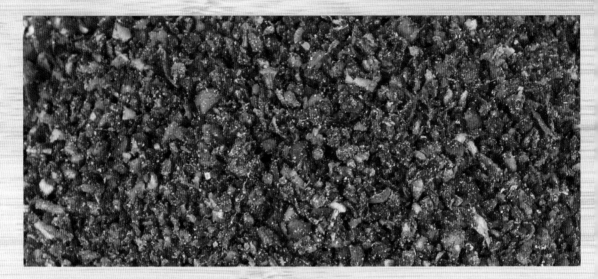

A member of the cashew and pistachio family, or *Anacardiaceae*, sumac refers to any of about 35 species of flowering plants. Grown all over the world, but most commonly found in East Asia, Africa, and parts of North America, these small shrubs and trees produce bright red fruits, or drupes, called sumac bobs. Some species produce drupes that are dried and ground to produce a flavorful—and colorful—spice. In fact, in the Syriac language, the word sumac means "red."

History and Use

This red spice, which has a tangy, lemony taste, is a staple in Middle Eastern and Arab cuisine, where it's added to salads, meat, hummus, and kebabs. Sumac is also used in the spice mixture za'atar, a popular condiment in the Middle East. As early as the 11th century, the spice was used not only for its flavor, but also for its medicinal benefits, being prescribed for fevers, asthma, stomach illnesses, and digestive imbalances. And pre-Columbian Native Americans used clusters of sumac drupes to create a refreshing beverage which they consumed as a healing tonic. Recipes for this tangy drink, now known as "sumac-ade" or "Indian lemonade," have become quite popular.

Health Benefits

Sumac's popularity is no wonder: the spice is high in vitamin C and is packed with antioxidants and antimicrobial compounds, providing it with healthy, plant-powered benefits. And research is backing up sumac's healing reputation, discovering that it may be beneficial for everything from diabetes to osteoporosis.

In one study, a group of participants with diabetes were given either three grams of sumac or a placebo daily over the course of three months. The group given the sumac were found to have decreased their blood sugar levels by 13 percent and improved their overall blood sugar regulation. Research has also shown that sumac may help to lower insulin levels and prevent insulin resistance.

Studies in animals have demonstrated that sumac is able to lower cholesterol and triglyceride levels, even in animals fed a high-cholesterol diet. The spice's heart-healthy high dose of antioxidants comes into play, as well, preventing heart disease and other chronic illnesses. These antioxidants also aid in reducing inflammation, which not only prevents disease but also helps to reduce pain. In fact, one study showed that adults who drank a juice made with sumac after aerobic exercise experienced less muscle soreness.

Fighting Bone Loss?

Sumac's natural antimicrobial properties have been used medicinally since medieval times. And modern studies have shown that the spice is effective in preventing the growth of many pathogens, including salmonella bacteria, which is responsible for many cases of food poisoning, and the fungus aspergillus, which can cause lung infections. But perhaps one of the most surprising benefits of this spice is its effect on bones: Sumac has been found to alter the balance of several proteins involved in bone metabolism, resulting in stronger bones and less bone loss. Although the studies are very new, the results are promising. Considering all of the proven benefits of this tasty spice, it certainly can't hurt to make it a regular part of your diet!

Ideas for Use

Sumac can be found in many grocery stores and Middle Eastern markets, or it can be purchased online. You can even buy bunches of drupes, and dry and grind the spice yourself, or use the berries to make homemade "sumac-ade." The lemony flavor of the spice works well in dressings, marinades, soups, vegetables, roasted meats, and salads, and many cooks prefer to sprinkle it on a dish just before serving, to add a pop of bright color and a tart flavor.

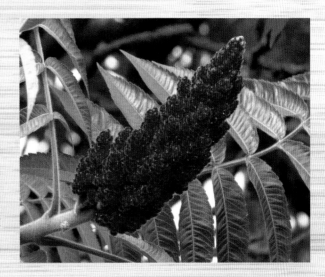

Vanilla

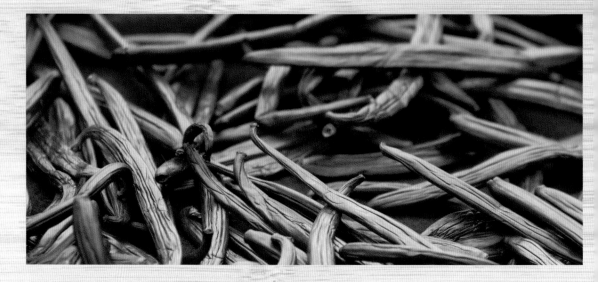

If you asked a roomful of people to name their favorite ice cream flavor, there's no doubt that vanilla would have quite a few votes. So it's no surprise that vanilla, with its instantly recognizable scent and distinctive flavor, is a hugely popular spice throughout the world. What may be surprising are the many health benefits that this sweet spice provides.

Origins

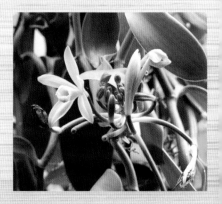

Vanilla is derived from orchids in the aptly named Vanilla genus. The three major species of vanilla orchids—grown today in Madagascar, the South Pacific, and in the West Indies and South and Central America—all originated in Mesoamerica, an area which includes modern-day Mexico. Until the 19th century, Mexico produced most of the vanilla in the world; but by the mid-1800s, merchants were shipping vanilla orchids to other parts of the world, in the hopes of creating their own vanilla crops.

There was a problem, however: the orchids required pollination in order to grow, but away from their native Mexico, no insects would pollinate the plants. Eventually, some of these orchids wound up on the French island of Réunion, where a 12-year-old slave named Edmond Albius created an ingenious technique for hand-pollinating the plants. This made the global cultivation of vanilla a profitable venture, and, in fact, Albius' hand-pollination technique is still used on vanilla orchids today.

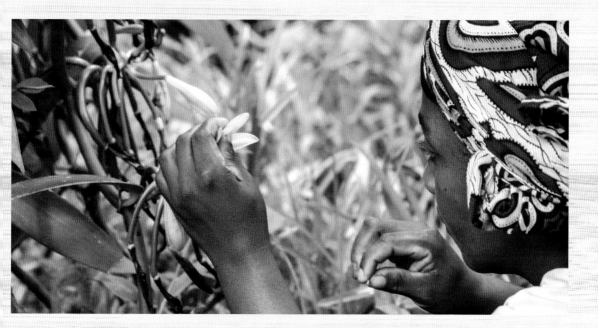

A Pricy Spice

Because of the amount of labor that goes into cultivating vanilla and the time it takes to produce the spice—it takes three years for a flower to produce one vanilla pod—it is the second-most expensive spice in the world, after saffron. But the cost doesn't seem to deter those who love this delectable spice.

Health Benefits

But vanilla is more than just a delicious flavoring for ice cream or a warm scent for perfume. The spice has some surprising health benefits, as well. Vanillin, one of the main compounds in vanilla, is an antioxidant that has been shown to reduce cholesterol levels in the body, preventing hardening of the arteries and blood clots. Research suggests that vanillin can reduce overall inflammation, lessening the symptoms of gout, arthritis and other inflammatory conditions. And there is some evidence that the spice may specifically provide protection for the liver, although studies are only at the preliminary stage.

Skin Saver

Vanilla also has antimicrobial properties that make it an effective tool against acne and other skin conditions. If used regularly, the spice can also reduce the appearance of previous acne scars and improve skin texture. And the skin-friendly benefits don't stop at acne. Experts also recommend using vanilla extract to reduce the inflammation of cold sores and speed healing. Simply soak a cotton ball in vanilla extract, and apply to the affected area several times a day until skin clears.

Baked Pumpkin Oatmeal

- 2 cups old-fashioned oats
- 2 cups milk
- 1 cup canned pumpkin
- 2 eggs
- ⅓ cup packed brown sugar
- 1 teaspoon vanilla
- ½ cup dried cranberries, plus additional for topping
- 1 teaspoon pumpkin pie spice
- ½ teaspoon salt
- ½ teaspoon baking powder
- Maple syrup
*** Chopped pecans (optional)

1. Preheat oven to 350°F. Spray 8-inch square baking dish with nonstick cooking spray.

2. Spread oats on ungreased baking sheet. Bake 10 minutes or until fragrant and lightly browned, stirring occasionally. Pour into medium bowl; let cool slightly.

3. Whisk milk, pumpkin, eggs, brown sugar and vanilla in large bowl until well blended. Add ½ cup cranberries, pumpkin pie spice, salt and baking powder to oats; mix well. Add oat mixture to pumpkin mixture; stir until well blended. Pour into prepared baking dish.

4. Bake 45 minutes or until set and knife inserted into center comes out almost clean. Serve warm with maple syrup, additional cranberries and pecans, if desired.

Makes 6 servings

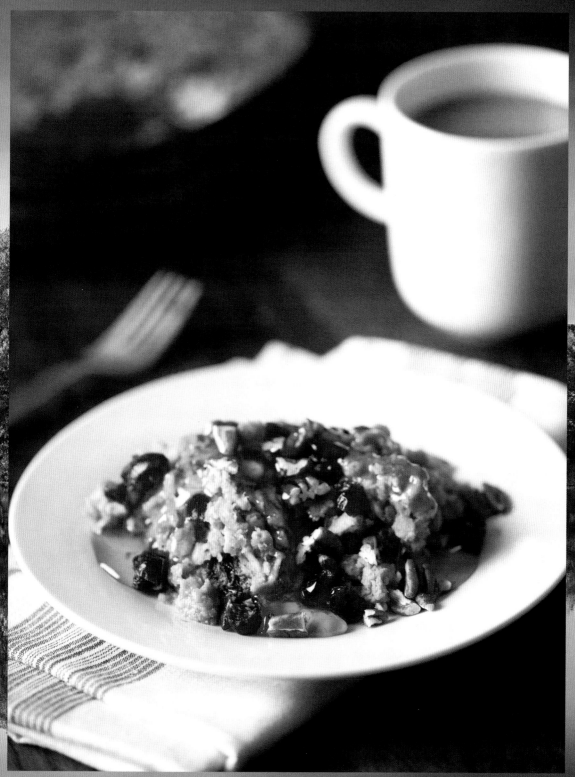

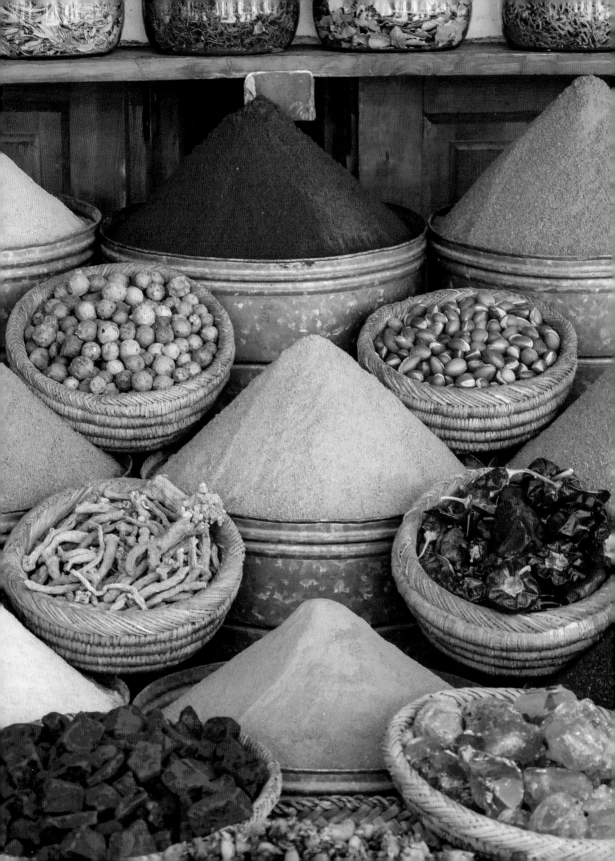